THE
Calcium LIE II

WHAT YOUR DOCTOR STILL DOESN'T KNOW

ROBERT THOMPSON, M.D. • KATHLEEN BARNES

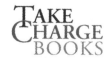
TAKE CHARGE BOOKS

Brevard, North Carolina

The purpose of the book is to educate. It is not intended to serve as a replacement for professional medical advice. Any use of this information in this book is at the reader's discretion. This book is sold with the understanding that neither the publisher nor the authors have any liability or responsibility for any injury caused or alleged to be caused directly or indirectly by the information contained in this book. While every effort has been made to ensure its accuracy, the book's contents should not be construed as medical advice. To obtain medical advice on your individual health needs, please consult a qualified health care practitioner.

Published by Take Charge Books
www.takechargebooks.com
e-mail: TakeChargeBooks2013@gmail.com

Library of Congress Cataloging-in-Publication Data

Thompson, Robert
Barnes, Kathleen
    The Calcium Lie II: What Your Doctor Still Doesn't Know
        p. cm.
    Includes bibliographic references and index.
    ISBN: 978-0-98838-665-5
    LCCN: 2013913861

Graphic design: Gary A. Rosenberg
Cover design: Brion Sausser, Book Creatives

Contents

Dedications

To my precious family, immediate and extended, I love you all.
Without your continued support and love, life becomes more difficult.
There are many ways to count our blessings. You bring much joy
and immeasurable wealth to each and every day of my life.

To my children, Nathan and Tiffany, it has been a privilege
beyond compare to watch you grow and to see you blossom.
I am proud to know you, let alone to call you my children.
Thank you for your love, your courage, and for making great
choices and living lives of distinction, character, integrity
and grandchildren. You make a dad smile.

To my patients and mentors for teaching me and challenging me
and to my Lord for the wisdom, blessings and salvation you have
given me. I am eternally grateful and thankful. May this book
bring honor and glory to your name through my life.

And to my sweet daughter-in-law, Cristin, and my son-in-law Cody, I
could not ask for a greater blessing of love for my beloved children. I
love you and your families with all my heart. I am proud to call you my
children-in-law. I am amazed and awe stricken that you are such perfect
and beautiful soul mates.

—DR. ROBERT THOMPSON

For Joe, as always,
with all my heart.

—KATHLEEN BARNES

Foreword

DR. ROBERT THOMPSON IS AN ENLIGHTENED PHYSICIAN.

His medical education gave him the knowledge of human physiology and biochemistry that he needed to become a competent physician. Dr. Thompson is among the elite, however, because his education did not end after graduation, but has continued throughout his career.

He became enlightened when he used his medical and scientific knowledge to surpass the knowledge of most other doctors, and formulated nutritional concepts based on basic scientific truths that are effective in treating and, dare I say, curing diseases that conventional medicine proclaims incurable.

Dr. Thompson is enlightened because of his unending dedication to helping his patients return to health and his passion for finding answers to his patients' health challenges.

Robert Thompson is a doctor in the true sense of the word. He is a teacher, as evidenced by his writings. Beyond all else, *The Calcium Lie* is intended to teach. Not only does this remarkable book teach about the intricate workings of the human body, it is also thought provoking.

The Calcium Lie can aid the average individual to understand and make sense of the complexities of the body in a down-to-earth fashion. This knowledge helps us to begin to ask questions about our health care rather than just accepting the status quo.

The Calcium Lie is a call to action to everyone who wants to become involved in and take responsibility for his own health.

Dr. Thompson's enlightenment is also demonstrated in the pioneering spirit of this book. The information contained herein is the wave of the future, because it teaches that we are individuals, and that therapeutic intervention should be based upon the individual need, and not merely a condition or disease process.

Dr. Thompson's viewpoint is certain to be controversial. It is my sincere hope that all readers, patients and physicians alike, carefully review the information offered here and recognize its value.

—David L. Watts, D.C. Ph.D., F.A.C.E.P.
CEO of Trace Elements, Inc., Addison, Texas

Introduction

WE ARE ALL VICTIMS OF HEALTH LIES. These lies, held with an almost religious zealotry, are quite literally killing us.

Primary among those lies is the notion that bones are made of calcium, with the dogmatic exhortation from almost every doctor on the planet that we all need supplemental calcium in order to have strong bones. This is absolutely untrue and without any reliable scientific evidence. In fact, our bones are made of at least 12 minerals, including calcium, and we need all of them in proper proportions in order to have healthy bones and a healthy metabolism. This is a "no brainer found in every biochemistry textbook, and yet we are all programmed to believe that we need calcium.

From this scientifically unfounded "get your calcium" supposition comes a cascade of health consequences that are nothing less than devastating. In this book, we will expose The Calcium Lie.

All research confirms our simple observation. It quite simply makes sense: We must abandon the notion that we cannot have strong bones without supplemental calcium. We must reveal the truth behind The Calcium Lie as quickly as possible, and begin to correct our mineral deficiencies and imbalances by replacing trace minerals with balanced trace minerals. Bones are made of minerals, not just calcium. Calcium hardens concrete!

You must know for certain your sodium, calcium and potassium levels and get expert advice about exactly which minerals to replace and in what amounts and which to avoid. All nutritional and medical recommendations without this information are fundamentally and scientifically flawed.

This is serious stuff. Much of our civilization and the health of future generations depend on it. Please do not underestimate the significance of these truths we describe to your long-term health. This is of paramount importance. Tell everyone you know and love to take minerals, not just calcium.

We've written and expanded this second edition of this book from a place of passionate conviction that our collective health is at risk from The Calcium Lie and a handful of other nutritional lies to which we are all subjected.

The truths in this second edition include an update of the original text with a few new and added thoughts, more detail, more bold statements, additional new references and a new chapter. We hope what you read here will lead you to a new life of exceptional health. That is anyone's most precious asset.

From Dr. Robert Thompson:

I am a caring doctor who went to medical school with altruistic ideas and a belief in doing the right thing and serving people. When I completed my medical training, I greeted my chosen career with great excitement about practicing medicine on the cutting edge, and doing the best job I could do for my patients.

Over the next few years, I grew increasingly disenchanted with my profession and with the uncharitable attitudes of many of my colleagues, who frequently resisted basic science and medical advances in the name of protecting their status quo. Even a local hospital where I worked was unhappy with me when some of my more advanced procedures (that included laparoscopic surgeries) resulted in outpatient, rather than inpatient, surgeries and shortened hospital stays. It really burst my idealistic new doctor bubble to learn that this hospital wanted its patients to stay in the hospital longer no matter what the trauma to the patient, because—"ca-ching"—the hospitals make more money that way. I guess I was just ahead of my time. Today, of course, outpatient surgery has become commonplace and routine as has laparoscopic surgery. For most of these procedures, the routine surgeries and profits are at an all-time high.

Finally, in 1996, I decided I was going to quit medicine. I was looking around for another career when I was notified I was chosen to be listed in an exclusive peer-reviewed directory, as one of the "Best Doctors in America."

I was overwhelmed by the honor, and the irony, that the honor came at a time when I had decided to hang up my stethoscope for good. Maybe all that training was not a waste after all. I took it as a sign that I was to remain in the medical profession and continue to try to make a difference.

I took it as a call back to my medical school training and ideals, and to some of the basic scientific concepts I seemed to have lost in the intervening years. That was an epiphany for me, and an opportunity for me to take a new look at the way I was treating my patients.

I realized that many of my pregnant patients were taking supplements and that, in order to be conscientious about their treatment, I needed to know more about them: what was good, what was bad, what worked, what didn't, and how much to take. I began to do more extensive research to find out which ones were safe for use in pregnancy and which ones weren't.

That opened new doors for me. I began learning about herbs, homeopathics and other natural treatments. I continued to grow and evolve in this process over the next few years, helping patients in new ways, often getting the same results—or sometimes even better—with natural treatments as with prescription drugs, but with less toxicity and fewer side effects.

I soon realized that I was still treating my patients' symptoms, perhaps with less toxicity, but nevertheless, like most doctors, I wasn't treating the underlying causes of their symptoms. I began to be more aware of the impact of nutrition in this equation. That opened new insights for me about the supplements people were taking, what was true about human nutrition and, more importantly, what was not true. Eventually, I discovered The Calcium Lie, The Vitamin Lie, The Sodium Lie, The Ascorbic Acid Lie, and other basic Nutritional Lies and I began to realize their impact on my patients' health and disease processes.

Along the way, I made many observations about what worked and what helped people get better and what didn't. As I continued to make recommendations to patients, I saw them continually getting better and overcoming their health problems, not just living with them. This is what we physicians were supposed to be doing all along. What a concept!

I was especially pleased to find ways to help my patients with type 2 diabetes and insulin resistance to overcome their blood sugar problems on a long-term basis. Were they "cured" of their diabetes? Maybe not, but what else can you call it when they have no symptoms and their laboratory tests and blood sugars remain in the normal range over many years?

I was tremendously excited about my discoveries. Unfortunately, I didn't find other caring physicians who shared my passion and were willing to listen to my ideas. Then I began attending meetings of the American College for Advancement in Medicine (ACAM) and the American Association of Anti-Aging Medicine (A4M), and another whole new medical world opened for me. In ACAM and A4M, I found like-minded doctors who realized there were better ways to treat patients, who were concerned about getting patients better and who were motivated to find and share them.

I'm not a zealot. I believe there are many good elements to conventional medicine. There are good medications, fantastic surgeries and cures and amazing advancements that were not available a decade or two ago. We don't need to "throw out the baby with the bathwater."

However, our current medical system is not only exorbitantly expensive, it has created a system in which doctors are reimbursed for allowing people to get sick rather than for keeping them healthy.

There is something fundamentally wrong with a system in which an insurance company will pay to amputate the leg of a diabetic patient rather than address prevention and healing with nutritional therapies and hyperbaric oxygen therapy—at less cost. This is a travesty of everything we stand for as physicians, as Americans and as caring people.

The medical profession as a whole has become greedy to a fault, compounded by exorbitant price gouging at every level. There is simply no reasonable excuse for some doctors making hundreds of thousand dollars and sometimes millions at the expense of the people they have been chosen to serve.

The hospitals (especially the "nonprofits"), the pharmaceutical and the medical technology industries have quite literally made health care unavailable to the average person. Even insurance companies have struggled to keep up with the exorbitant prices. The system is broken at almost every level. Maybe we should require all physicians to get a salary like those who serve our military based on rank and level of training. Something has to change. Too many people are suffering.

The lack of accountability for poor results has been largely overlooked in the medical profession of the U.S. The United States is now 46th in men's mortality with life expectancy of around 76 years, 47th in women's mortality with life expectancy of 80 years, and the U.S. has dropped to 34th in the world in infant mortality, a drop from 23rd ten years ago. In spite of all our high-risk obstetrics and perinatal care and all the new technology, specialists and perinatal care, the U.S. is the absolute *worst* country in the industrialized world in first-day infant mortality.

If our seniors make it to 85 years of age, they have a 50 percent chance of having dementia and not knowing it. Even more worrisome, there has been an increase in maternal death in childbirth in the last decade for the first time in 50 years. We are also among the worst in the world in preterm births with 1 in 8 babies born before full term.

Nearly every disease is increasing:

- Based on the current rate of increase in autism, there will be *no* normal male babies born in the U.S. by 2030.

- The current rate of diabetes increase suggests that the diseased will have stricken 95 percent of our adult population by 2030.

- Autoimmune disease now affects over 150 million of our citizens and increases every year.

- The number of children with life-threatening allergies has increased over 1000 percent.

- Toxic superbug bacteria are literally eating us alive.

- Cancer keeps increasing in frequency every decade unabated by our medical profession or its leadership, which seems to be stuck in protecting the status quo, the Almighty Dollar. Just look at the exquisite facilities for the treatment of cancer patients, all the new buildings, all the incredible technology for treating this disease, the expensive experimental drugs, the multimillion dollar radiation therapy centers, and we easily see, cancer is big business. Cancer now affects nearly 50 percent of our population as does heart and vascular disease.

These are just a few of the most important health problems we face.

Obviously, our health is important to us. Our drug company-driven health care industry in the U.S. spends more than three times as much on our health care as any other developed country in the world (not including nutritional supplements) for what I would consider dismal and embarrassing results.

These statistics do not lie. They keep getting worse. That alone should be a clue we are going in the wrong direction. Health care costs in the U.S. are over $2.8 trillion and increasing every year. This is big business! It is nearly five times what we spend on our national defense.

Unfortunately, the nutrition industry also has its flaws. Its focus is largely about sales. It is quite similar to the pharmaceutical industry in many respects, but once again, there are some amazingly effective supplements on the market today.

Physicians need to educate themselves about nutrition and learn to make a real difference in their health and their patient's health before it is too late. First, physicians must truly care. Rarely does the all-too-frequent commercial admonition to "ask your doctor" really get an educated answer. More often, it gets an uninformed attitude or belief espoused with ignorant arrogance. The physician most often remains ignorant about these matters by choice.

Supplements can produce good results for you if you take the right ones. There is also tremendous waste here. Exorbitant amounts of money are spent on supplements that have little or no nutritional value or health benefit. Even more important, the best supplement in the world will not be as effective or will not work at all if the basic nutritional needs as outlined in this book are not being addressed or are being done so incorrectly.

I realized that, just as I would try to pick out the best medication for treating a medical problem, I needed to be accountable for trying to help my patients pick out the best supplements to make up for the tremendous nutritional deficiencies in our food and to do so in ways that change our health for the better and in ways that are measurable. Most patients would prefer that their doctors discover and treat the underlying causes of their disease rather than treating the symptoms. Unfortunately, some patients just want a pill to treat their symptoms; they are not really motivated to get better. Being healthy is a choice and a responsibility, not a right.

Your health is your most valuable asset. Obviously it is important to us, we spend exorbitantly on it. But we must take accountability for our results, which at this juncture are quite dismal. We must begin to apply the preventative information we know, and as presented in this book.

To keep doing the same things and expecting different results is insanity. To accept the current downward health trends is just plain unacceptable.

In the end, patients and physicians are going to have to realize that withholding care and rationing of care are likely to become commonplace because, as a society, we simply cannot afford to pay for all the health crises we are developing as our population ages. We must change our collective health now to decrease our future costs in financial and personal terms. We must carefully protect ourselves as best we can from nutritional deficiencies, imbalances and toxins or suffer from ever worsening health statistics.

Colleagues and patients began to encourage me to write this book more than six years before the first edition of *The Calcium Lie* was published.

This message is so important, that it has caused the book to keep increasing in sales without an agent, without public appearances, without anything except an important message spreading from person to person.

Now, here comes the second edition. As in the first edition, I am putting this information out there for patients and physicians alike to learn from it and grow into greater health awareness. There are many books out there; however, we believe this one is unique and profound. Since our first edition, an increasing body of research has confirmed almost every claim we have made. Much of the information we discuss has already existed as fact in various references, but has apparently been ignored. This book puts the most important of these facts together. It literally "connects the dots."

The impact of *The Calcium Lie II* (as was the first edition, *The Calcium Lie*) is *huge* in terms of its potential impact on health care worldwide, now and in the future. Reversing many long-held beliefs, it represents fundamental changes in medical practice recommendations that can't take place fast enough.

To the best of our ability, we have made an attempt to provide truth, facts and reliable information in simple terms, and in ways the average person can understand.

My coauthor, Kathleen Barnes, and I have written this book together, although much of it is in first person based on my experience.

Kathleen Barnes is a health journalist with great depth of experience, not only in conventional medical research and terminology, but through the passion she has had for natural health for more than 30 years. She is author or editor of 20 books, most of them on natural health subjects, and she wrote a weekly natural health column for *Woman's World* magazine for more than six years.

Her ability to help translate complex medical terminology into simple and easily understandable terms has helped me to stay on the "straight and narrow" when I tend to get too technical in my concepts.

If you've read this book and it resonates with you, tell a friend. Give a copy to a friend. You may be saving a life.

We invite you to copy the last chapter of this book and give it to your doctor, with our blessing. Better yet, buy a copy as a gift for your doctor. You and your fellow patients will reap the benefits if your doctor can be persuaded to invest the few hours it takes to read this book.

We wish you all the best in your quest to maintain and regain your health. If you apply the principles in this book, we have no doubt you will succeed.

—Robert Thompson, M.D., Soldotna, Alaska
—Kathleen Barnes, Brevard, North Carolina

CHAPTER 1

Minerally Bankrupt

THERE'S A BIG LIE THAT HAS SUCKED US ALL IN, consumers and medical professionals alike. That Big Lie is killing us.

What's the lie?

It started with a wild notion that calcium is essential for strong bones. Nearly all of our doctors and most of us have bought into this "Calcium Lie," hook, line and sinker. We were all led to believe that unless we get loads of calcium, our bones will break and crumble to powder. It's not true. It's never been true and basic science taught in every university in the world shows us the error of this belief system.

Before we go any further, let us tell you that calcium is only one of at least 12 minerals that build strong bones.

If you take calcium to strengthen your bones and you already have an excess of calcium in your body, you are signing your own death warrant. Think of it like this: **Calcium hardens concrete.** Imagine what it can harden in your body! Excess calcium can cause:

- Kidney and gallstones

- Arterial plaque

- Bone spurs

- Calcium deposits in tissues other than bones

- Brain cell dysfunction, brain shrinkage and dementia

The story behind The Calcium Lie

What caused us to buy into The Calcium Lie and how are we paying for the error of our ways? Here's the story:

The invention of the refrigerator was the beginning of humankind's modern health crisis.

In 1876, the first practical refrigerator was invented and refrigerators became commonly available by the turn of the century.

So why did this cause a health crisis for humankind?

The answer is simple: We stopped using sea or rock salt to preserve our meat and other foods. We thereby robbed our bodies of the essential minerals in that salt that we need to survive and thrive (sea salt contains perfectly balanced ionic trace minerals). And henceforth, generation after generation has experienced declining tissue mineral levels.

Medical science has flourished in the past century with advances ranging from the invention of synthetic insulin to antibiotics to CAT scans, MRIs, robotic surgery, joint replacement and many more technical advances.

These medical miracles may all have their places, but without the basic building blocks of nutrition that we need to maintain, sustain and repair our bodies, we humans are never going to find the vibrant health that should be our birthright.

At the moment, this is a squandered birthright. However, we can begin to regain our health by simple and affordable nutritional means. In the process, we can reduce, successfully treat and even eliminate some of the greatest health challenges of our time including: obesity, diabetes, cancer, atherosclerosis (hardening of the arteries and heart disease), hypertension, hypothyroidism, osteoporosis, depression, migraines, dementia, many autoimmune diseases and many more illnesses

How? The answer is so simple it will surprise you.

All we have to do is add back minerals into our diets daily in the forms of natural sea salt or rock salt and ionic balanced trace mineral supplements. We need to add minerals to our food and use them in supplemental form. We desperately need to put trace minerals back into our bodies every day, every way we can, from now on for the rest of our lives.

We must begin immediate and specific corrections of the mineral levels that are already out of balance based on reliable scientific measurement.

The best form of this measurement is by reliable HTMA (hair tissue mineral analysis).

We also must begin to use whole-food vitamins only along with the correct minerals for individual needs. Minerals and whole-food vitamins are the basics. Without these basics, nothing else really matters.

A little painless biochemistry

Please bear with us for a few paragraphs while we review with you the basic science that underlies this astonishing shortsightedness on the part of humankind and specifically on the part of the medical profession. We have all failed to understand and recognize the importance of the basic biochemistry that lies at the heart of the medical conditions that plague modern humans.

You probably already know that our bodies are mainly water. On the average, 72 percent of your body weight is water, pure and simple. If you weigh 150 pounds, you have 108 pounds of water in your body. This is a basic premise of our physiology: Anything we put in our bodies MU.S.T be water-soluble or have a specific transport mechanism to be absorbed.

The remainder of your body weight is minerals: all 28 percent of it. For a 150-pound person, this means you're carrying around 42 pounds of a life-giving soup of 76 ionizing essential and trace minerals, ranging from the commonly known calcium, magnesium, sodium and potassium to the more esoteric chromium, manganese, selenium and copper, to the more rare trace minerals like lithium, rubidium, cobalt, germanium and molybdenum, to name a few.

Bear with us. This is getting exciting.

Now, the planet's oceans and salt beds contain *all* of the minerals and trace minerals we need to be in perfect health.

True sea salt and rock salt contain all of the minerals in the *exact* proportion that our bodies require (except sodium; more about that later). Quite simply, these minerals are necessary for every single body function to work: biochemical, electrical, chemical and physiological.

We don't know about you, but we find this awe inspiring, miraculous and perhaps one of the strongest scientific arguments for the existence of an intelligent creative force that is beyond our comprehension.

We're going minerally downhill

Getting back to the refrigerator, when we stopped preserving our food with naturally occurring sea salts, we became progressively deficient in some, if not all, of those essential minerals. Because a mineral "fingerprint" is passed from mother to child (more about that in Chapter 6), each generation has become progressively more deficient in these essential minerals.

At about the same time salt was "purified," humankind in all of its wisdom began to severely deplete the soil in which we grow our food. The introduction of chemical fertilizers actually further robbed and depleted the soil of its nutrients.

We also began to build huge dams to control and reduce natural flooding. We might think that this was a good idea, but it wasn't necessarily so, since floodwaters actually carry essential mineral nutrients back into the land. Plants grown in these mineral-poor soils were increasingly unable to extract the nutrients into their produce and bring them to our tables. Without certain specific minerals, vitamins cannot be formed (more about that in Chapter 7). In short, vitamins cannot be produced or work without minerals.

In 1936, the U.S. Senate actually warned the population that our soil was seriously depleted of minerals. The warning was based on research from such prestigious academic institutions as Yale, Rutgers, Johns Hopkins and Columbia in conjunction with the U.S. Department of Agriculture.

Dr. Charles Northern, one of the lead researchers in these projects, issued a prophetic warning at the time: " . . . Countless human ills stem from the fact that the impoverished soil of America no longer provides plant foods with mineral elements essential to human nourishment and health. Millions of acres no longer contain the valuable trace elements . . . It is not commonly realized, however, that vitamins control the body's appropriation of minerals, and in the absence of minerals they have no function to perform. Lacking vitamins, the system can make some use of minerals, but lacking minerals, vitamins are useless."

Decades later, Dr. Northern's warning was underscored by Dr. Linus Pauling, winner of two Nobel prizes, who is credited with saying, "You can trace every sickness, every disease and every ailment to a mineral deficiency."

Clearly the warnings fell on deaf ears.

Since then, the problem has gotten worse. A 1992 Earth Summit report placed the decline in mineral content of North American soils at 85 percent and seven years later, in 1999, a Rutgers University study revealed the mineral content of commercial fruits and vegetables was less than 16 percent of normal compared to vine-ripened organic produce, and the trace elements necessary for vitamin production were completely absent. Since the mineral content determines the vitamin content, our commercial produce has almost no nutritional value! As you will hear repeatedly in this book, we have to supplement our food and do so correctly in order to be healthy.

It's no wonder that we are sick when we take into account the facts that much of our produce has often been shipped thousands of miles, picked before prime ripeness, grown in nutrient-deficient soil and loses nutrients during shipping.

Organic foods *may* have lower levels of organophosphates (pesticides and herbicides), but no increased nutritional value unless they are vine ripened. We'll go into the benefits of vine-ripened and organic foods in coming chapters, but it's important to know now that the mineral content of vine-ripened fruits and vegetables is substantially higher than that of commercially produced foods, so get vine-ripened, fresh, raw, unheated, fresh frozen or dried fruits and vegetables and go organic as much as you can! In winter, you can get some of your needs from raw nuts and seeds, but it will almost certainly be necessary for you to take a balanced ionic trace mineral supplement and the real vitamin C (not as ascorbic acid).

Mineral disruptors

Bromine is another serious issue in terms of food and medicine. Bromine has been implicated in thyroid disease and cancer, breast cysts, fibrous changes, cyclic tenderness and cancer, prostate inflammation and cancer, pancreatic dysfunction and cancer, and ovarian hormonal dysfunction, ovarian cysts, endometriosis and ovarian cancer. These problems have been attributed to the bromine's interference with iodine functions, which most severely affects the endocrine gland system.

Bromine has been added to our flour for over 30 years (except King

Arthur brand flour and a few others). Bromine as methyl bromide is also sprayed on our fruits to stop mold from growing, especially on berries, and it cannot be washed off. It is added to many canned foods, bottled foods, carbonated drinks, energy drinks and bakery products as a leavening agent and as a food preservative. Bromine is also often used in swimming pools and spas to kill bacteria instead of the more volatile less toxic chlorine (chlorine evaporates faster).

Animal studies have shown that hypothyroidism (low thyroid function) is a result of eating foods containing bromine. Worse yet, the toxicity of bromine is increased in pregnant women, so be particularly careful if you are pregnant or planning on becoming pregnant.

The U.S. Department of Agriculture (USDA) mandated the addition of bromine to flour in 1980 despite the fact that bromine has been shown to cause apathy, decreased concentration, depression, headaches, irritability, delirium, schizophrenia, psychomotor retardation and hallucinations as well as the endocrine cancers as suggested above.

The only antidote for bromine is increased iodine intake and increased intake of chloride as sodium chloride (salt). The kidneys have a difficult time in eliminating bromine when the body is deficient in sodium chloride, which extends the time it takes to eliminate the bromine by more than 800 percent in laboratory animals.

Table salt is a health destroyer

Then came the final blow: Early in the 20th century, more "scientific" advances brought us pretty, white, convenient table salt that was composed only of two minerals: sodium and chloride or sodium chloride. It was a fine and granular salt. It was convenient and didn't clump in humidity like sea salt. Scientists of the time apparently considered the other 74 ionizing minerals present in rock salt and sea salt to be unnecessary, unsightly and inconvenient due to humidity causing clumping, so they were "purified" out.

The result: The first evidence of our grave error came in 1924 when we began to see iodine deficiency within our population leading to the widespread development of thyroid goiter and increasing mental retardation (enlargement of the thyroid gland and thyroid hormone deficiency and "cretinism"). This led to the addition of another mineral to sodium chloride, as potassium iodide or iodine, and our pretty white table salt became "iodized salt." This should have been our first clue that many other vital nutrients were missing. But we failed to recognize the signals. Our collective downhill slide into widespread mineral deficiency began to accelerate.

Our bodies began to desperately seek the minerals we need to survive, to the point where they even drew on similar-acting minerals to try to duplicate the missing nutrients, actually substituting for the minerals needed. This is the Thompson-Döbereiner principle of mineral substitution. (See Chapter 3)

The Calcium Lie in brief

The Mineral Lie was the first of many lies. The Calcium Lie, which is an outgrowth of the Mineral Lie, has led us to a host of health problems of untold proportions. We'll go into them in greater detail in the coming chapters, but here is the foundation of The Calcium Lie:

Most people, even many medical professionals, began to believe that bones are made of calcium. As we've said before, our bones are actually composed of at least 12 minerals. One of them is calcium, but a proper balance of all these minerals is essential for bone health, strong bones and the prevention of osteoporosis. By the way, osteoporosis is defined as a loss of minerals from the bones, not a loss of just calcium. Remember, calcium hardens concrete, not bones!

Our doctors told us we needed more calcium to keep our bones strong, so we started popping calcium supplements, adding calcium to many of our foods and we were told to drink at least two glasses of calcium-rich milk every day. This false belief also commonly leads nondairy consuming individuals to "fortify" with extra calcium in their diet.

This gross oversimplification for the apparent benefit of the dairy industry's (The Dairy "Get Your Calcium" Lie) is similar to The Mineral Lie, The Vitamin Lie (Chapter 7) and the Iodine Story. What we've sacrificed in the name of simplification and convenience has led us to serious errors and the propagation of outright lies in an approach to health that has taken a devastating toll.

Ask yourself, what are your bones made of? What builds strong bones?

What is osteoporosis, a loss of what from the bones? Almost everyone, including educated medical personnel, dieticians and even physicians, will all answer, "Calcium." That's The Calcium Lie.

This is a big mistake! We are so programmed to believe that our bones are made of calcium, that it has almost become dogmatic.

Here's the truth: If you take calcium supplements and eat calcium-rich foods (probably on the recommendation of your doctor), you'll build up excess calcium in your system coupled with increasing mineral deficiencies and imbalances that will help cause plaque in arteries, kidney stones, gall-stones, bone spurs, osteoarthritis, hypertension (high blood pressure), thyroid hormone resistance or what I have correctly described as type 2 hypothyroidism, obesity, type 2 diabetes, brain shrinkage and dementia and many other diseases we'll address in this book.

When we took the unrefined salts like sea salt and rock salt out of our diets, we lost about 15 percent of the nutritional value of our foods.

Incorrect suggestions to limit sodium intake, even as sea salt, increased our mineral deficiencies. Adding calcium to our diets to try to correct multiple mineral deficiencies and prevent or treat osteoporosis won't help. This is a failed and incorrect hypothesis. Taking calcium alone will actually make our mineral imbalances worse. Excess calcium causes more mineral deficiencies and creates mineral imbalances leading to a downward spiral of numerous medical problems.

In addition, calcium doesn't significantly improve fracture risks from osteoporosis and calcium excess leads to a myriad of other nutritional problems, including nutrient digestion and absorption issues and multiple diseases.

Our belief that calcium is the essential element for strong bones is an erroneous idea that has turned into an outright lie. Today nearly all of us believe we need extra calcium to have healthy bones and to prevent osteoporosis. More is better, so we add calcium. It is added to everything from orange juice to sports drinks, cereal, baby food, soy-based drinks and pasta. The list is endless.

We need minerals. We need *all* of them, not just one mineral.

Worst of all, we feed our children calcium-rich milk in the mistaken belief it will give them strong bones. By doing this we are subjecting them to hardening of the arteries later in life, hypothyroidism, hypoadrenalism,

From Dr. Thompson

Over the last 18 years, I have continually been faced with The Calcium Lie. Lay folks can be forgiven for their ignorance of biochemistry, but it is appalling when I encounter physicians and dieticians who hold the same disastrous misconception. In fact, I've repeatedly encountered doctors who tell me they are going to continue to recommend calcium and the calcium-elevating hormone vitamin D to their patients, even after they are reminded of the basic biochemistry of our bodies. They doggedly go back to what they want to believe.

This is what the drug company-sponsored research, public advertising and the dairy industry have preached to us with a religious fervor. This is programming personified, intellectual dishonesty or just downright ignorance. Could these so-called protectors of our health be practicing a religion, not a science? To ignore these basic facts, after one is made aware of them, is most certainly intellectual dishonesty.

The medical profession must abandon the error of recommending calcium without knowing if it is warranted.

"Get your Calcium" is a failed hypothesis. Bones are quite simply not made of calcium alone. Calcium should no longer be considered the treatment for osteoporosis. We must replace our mineral deficiencies with balanced ionic trace minerals.

In the process of completing a medical education, the average physician has taken at least four six-hour courses in chemistry, organic chemistry and biochemistry. This is sufficient for every single one of them to understand far more than the essentials of biochemistry and human physiology. But for some reason, doctors choose to be programmed, to quit thinking, to conveniently "forget" or simply not to absorb these scientific truths. Could it be that their own mineral deficiencies have affected their thought processes or their backbones?

Of course, I'm being a little facetious here, but The Calcium Lie is the result of selective and misleading advertising and biased and flawed research that has deceived our country and our medical professionals and the world.

Two "prominent" physicians at a hospital where I worked attacked me over the first edition of this book and did so admittedly without reading it and without examining a single reference. This is a sad, but true story. They chose to remain ignorant and to maintain their false beliefs, all the while disparaging me personally for speaking out and disagreeing with me without knowing what it was specifically that they were disagreeing with. This is truly shameful.

The cost of The Calcium Lie has been enormous. It has cost us our health and that of the coming generations.

> I am amazed at the degree of mineral deficiency in our populations all across the earth. I now have patients from Australia to the Netherlands and everywhere in between, so I know these mineral deficiencies and imbalances are worldwide. Today, it's worse than ever in our younger populations. Yet, the American government and many of its "intelligent" organizations and agencies still push the idea that we all need one to two servings of dairy products or a calcium supplement every day.
>
> About 90 percent of us do not need any extra dietary calcium at all! Since dairy products are the major sources of dietary calcium in the Standard American Diet (SAD for short), this opens the dairy industry to suspicion.
>
> When will we ever forget our programming? Please press the "delete" button in your mind, erase the calcium obsession and replace it with the idea that minerals are your body's greatest need, after its need for pure water.
>
> My goal is that, after reading this book, at a minimum you will stop taking calcium supplements and start taking balanced ionic trace minerals and spread the message as fast as possible to those you love and care about.

autoimmune disease, allergies and even obesity. We can all give thanks to the dairy industry's advertising for that lie.

The U.S. government, our research institutions and most of all our doctors, should have instantly grasped this simple biochemical truth: Too much calcium causes an imbalance of minerals in the body. This leads to an accumulation of calcium in the tissues. This calcium excess not only causes huge changes in our intercellular (between the cells) metabolism, but it also leads to calcium deposits in the intracellular (inside the cell) spaces. These calcium deposits form gravel-like plaque throughout our arteries, kidney stones, gallstones and joint deterioration. Excess calcium also accelerates brain aging and causes impaired memory, brain shrinkage and dementia.

Yes, we do need some calcium. For most people, the calcium in balanced ionic trace minerals is totally adequate and scientifically correct. Yes, calcium is still important, but most of us get far too much of it. This imbalance is causing us to take more medications in order to treat the mineral deficiency-related diseases caused by these mineral imbalances. This includes increases in all diseases of aging, cancer, stroke, type 2 diabetes, obesity, metabolic syndrome, type 2 hypothyroidism, depression, anxiety, insomnia, migraines, circulatory diseases, hypertension, heart disease, immune compromise, dementia and many more health problems.

What are we doing? We are slowly turning ourselves into concrete statues. Remember, calcium hardens concrete!

Why have we been victimized by this illogical thinking? Is it false and unscrupulous advertising, a vast conspiracy, special interest lobbying groups, capitalism gone awry or government complacency? We have no answers to these important questions, but our current national state of health is living (or perhaps dying) proof that this has happened to our collective psyche. The proof is in the pudding. We believe rational and intellectually honest humans can deduce the truth and realize the error of the "get your calcium" message.

We simply must change this message to "get your trace minerals."

Calcium and adrenal gland function

Here comes some more biochemistry. Please bear with us!

Too much calcium causes the adrenal glands to be suppressed in order for the kidneys to hold on to the necessary magnesium in an attempt to keep these two minerals in balance. This adrenal suppression results in sodium and potassium being continuously excreted into the urine in large amounts, draining intracellular stores of these important minerals, even though our bodies are desperately seeking additional sources of these two essential minerals. Sodium is needed for stomach acid production, protein digestion, for facilitating transfer of glucose and amino acids into the cells of all our organs and tissues, except fat cells. Potassium is essential for thyroid hormone function and helps maintain cell membrane electrical potential.

These essential minerals are critical to ensure a steady heartbeat so that muscle and nerve fibers will fire when they are needed. They also insure that blood pressure remains stable. It is my contention that most all atrial fibrillation (commonly called Afib) is caused by or directly related to these chronic mineral imbalances and deficiencies. These mineral deficiencies and imbalances lead to electrical failure in the electrical conduction cells of the heart. It can be induced over time by depriving these cells of minerals with bisphosphonate drugs used to treat osteoporosis. Over time, these drugs can cause Afib as a downstream effect from robbing the body and especially the heart of the mineral stores it needs because the needed minerals are being kept in the bone. This problem can be prevented with adequate balanced trace mineral replacements that will help correct the imbalances and prevent the deficiencies.

Excess calcium and the resulting deficiencies in sodium and potassium cause a failure of the cell membrane electrical potential (CMEP) and this severely limits energy production in the cells with far-reaching health consequences. The calcium, potassium, sodium and magnesium balance inside and outside our cells is critical to life and health and is maintained by this electrical potential at the cell membrane.

Specialized pores in the cell membrane help move potassium into the cells, where it is bound to the protein molecules imbedded in the cell membrane. Sodium is moved out of cells, and potassium into the cells, with the help of a microscopic electrical charge. This same electrical "pumping" mechanism that moves sodium out of the cells brings glucose, amino acids and other nutrients into every cell in our bodies along with sodium, except fat cells, which absorb glucose directly without the help sodium.

It's not hard to imagine what happens when there is not enough sodium and potassium to create this electrical membrane pumping system. The body's ability to get amino acids and glucose into all its cells is severely limited (except fat cells, which still absorb glucose and continue to grow). This electrical potential membrane failure causes many other cellular metabolic failures that have long-reaching consequences. Without these amino acids, your body cannot grow and repair itself. Without glucose, your cells have no fuel for energy. We must have electrons donated by minerals for every biochemical reaction that takes place in our cells. Thus mineral deficiency creates serious consequences for your health and your whole body.

In my practice, I've discovered that the average patient has only 7.5 to 15 percent of the normal intracellular sodium and potassium content in spite of blood tests that show "normal" levels. That's why I tell patients with confidence, based on tissue mineral analysis results, that they are making a big mistake when they boast that they "hardly eat any salt." I call this The Sodium Lie. More than 90 percent of us need *more* sodium. Only testing can tell you for sure.

Go ionic

If you are adding supplemental minerals to your regimen, be sure they are balanced ionic minerals. These are the only ones that are water soluble in your water-based body. They are the only types of minerals with an electrical charge that allows them to move freely into the cells where they can participate in beneficial cell function and help to maintain the all-important cell membrane electrical potential. (More about this in Chapter 4.)

In the presence of enzymes, ionic minerals allow trillions of chemical reactions to take place in our bodies every second, at a relatively neutral pH of 7.4, and a consistent temperature of 98.6 degrees Fahrenheit. This is quite simply a miracle.

Ionic minerals are the most plentiful form of minerals found on earth. They are found in all fresh water, inground deposits in places where oceans once existed and, of course, in the oceans themselves. All fresh water tables on earth have specific fingerprints of approximately 55 ionic minerals.

Fresh water makes its way to the ocean through a wide variety of mineral strata. As our water finds its way to the sea, it continues to pick up minerals, eventually forming the great rivers that empty into our oceans, which are the world's "great mixing pot" of all ionic minerals in salt form. These oceans (and sea salt deposits from dried ocean beds), by some miracle, contain a supersaturated solution of all the minerals found in mammals and humans in the perfect balance and concentrations we need for good health, except sodium. (More about that later.) Sea salt has all the ionic minerals and trace minerals we need for good health.

You may have heard of colloidal minerals. Some misinformed people have pushed them as the be-all and end-all of human nutrition. They are dead wrong. You will be too, if you listen to them.

Think about minerals like iron or copper or even chalk-like calcium. How can you get these heavy molecules into your body?

It's time for another painless biochemistry lesson.
Remember what we said earlier about your body being 72 percent water? The *only* way for your body to absorb and use minerals is for them to dissolve in water with an electrical charge, in other words, to become ionic. It is simple science. No matter how much a mineral may be mixed, pulverized and powdered, or derived from decayed plant materials (sometimes called

colloidal minerals), which by definition don't dissolve, don't conduct electricity and don't cross cell membranes easily if at all, it can't be absorbed. There is no way on God's green earth that your body can use this form of mineral effectively.

These solids and suspensions, no matter how small they are, cannot pass through cell membranes or conduct electricity, so they are of no use to the body.

In fact, colloidal minerals can even be harmful because their mineral residues can end up in between your cells, or in your bloodstream, clogging up things and generally getting in the way. Eventually, these mineral residues become permanently deposited between the cells, causing inflammation, cell compression, peripheral vascular disease, atherosclerosis, heart disease and stroke. That's how these substances escalate the disease processes they are touted to treat.

The best example of these harmful mineral supplements is colloidal silver, which over time will accumulate permanently between your cells, including the skin, causing it to look black or tarnished (the oxidation process of silver). These so-called "nutritional supplements" simply don't dissolve, don't conduct electricity, don't cross semipermeable membranes and their byproducts have to accumulate somewhere. Their internal use should be completely abandoned or prohibited in humans.

Never, ever, take colloidal minerals! There is simply no real benefit and significant potential for harm.

You may also have heard of chelated minerals. These types of fine mineral powders bonded with amino acids do have their place. They do allow varied amounts of absorption. Chelated minerals can be important when a specific individual mineral deficiency has been identified and needs to be corrected. Routinely taking vitamins or supplements that contain chelated minerals, however, may cause problems, especially if those specific minerals are already in excess in the body. So, you still need to have a hair tissue mineral analysis (HTMA) to be sure the product or supplement contains what you need and won't create further excesses. Almost any mineral can be harmful or dangerous if it is taken in excess.

Did you ever notice that your sweat and your tears taste like salt? We lose salty minerals through our sweat and urine every day. Therefore, we clearly need to replace our mineral supply daily.

Hair Tissue Mineral Analysis (HTMA)

A quick word about HTMA: Human hair tissue is particularly useful to identify specific mineral levels, deficiencies and imbalances because hair is easy to obtain and is the most convenient. With correct sampling, it is a simple and highly accurate way to test tissue mineral levels by utilizing the science of micro-mass spectrophotometry. Hair grows from the inside to the outside of the cell, so it accurately reflects the intracellular mineral content of our bodies. Over 95 percent of all the minerals in the body are intracellular, so hair is an extremely valuable diagnostic tool.

Getting an HTMA test from a reputable and reliable Clinical Laboratory Improvement Amendments (CLIA) certified lab is essential to knowing your personal mineral profile, your unique needs and your imbalances. This test quite simply may be the most important health test of all known to medical science. Unfortunately, the medical profession has often taken an ignorant approach to this test and its science. While certain variations occur with HTMA results for very specific reasons, the test is highly reliable and reproducible.

Replace your lost minerals with ionic (salt form) minerals and find your way back to health. There is no need to restrict your sea salt intake unless you have had a hair tissue mineral analysis that specifically shows excess sodium in your cells, which is less than 10 percent of all results.

Long-lived cultures

So what's the evidence for these mineral truths?

Aside from the logic of basic biochemistry that most seventh graders can understand and certainly any college freshman can assimilate, we offer the proof of the longest-lived cultures on earth.

There are many similarities between these seemingly diverse cultures: the Tibetans in China's northeast plateau, the Hunzas in Pakistan, the Titicacans of Peru's Andes Mountains, the Vilacamba of the Ecuadorean Andes and the Russian Georgians and their sister cultures, the Abkhazians, Azerbaijanis and the Armenians of the Caucasus mountains as far as northern Turkey. Centenarians, those who live more than 100 years, are quite common in these cultures.

The large amount of sea salt consumption (up to 20 grams per day in some cases) and longevity in these simple cultures is a strong indicator of the value of minerals from natural salts, either from the seas or from the salt mines that mark the remains of ancient seas. It's something our society should reconsider. Industrialization clearly isn't always progress. While I am not necessarily advocating this large amount of sea salt consumption, it is the basis for my recommendation that almost everyone needs 3 grams of essential balanced trace minerals per day.

The modern-day Okinawans are another remarkable example of long life, according to the Okinawa Centenarian Study. The study says Okinawa has 50 centenarians for every 100,000 islanders, the highest ratio in the world. The United States has between 10 and 20 centenarians for every 100,000 people—about one-third of the number of really old folks as in Okinawa. Life expectancy is 81.2 years on Okinawa, the longest in the world. New figures show that the average Okinawan woman lives to 86 and the average man to 78.

Okinawans don't just live longer, they live better, says a 2002 article in *U.S. Today.* "According to recent studies, the elderly here appear to have far lower rates of dementia than their U.S. counterparts and suffer less than half the risk for hip fractures. Some Okinawan centenarians even claim they are still having sex." Some researchers aren't so sure about that. Personally, we hope it is true!

Many of these long-lived people are from comparatively primitive agrarian cultures. Most of them live at higher elevations, and habitually they eat large quantities of sea salt from mined salt rich in *all* minerals from local deposits of the long-dried beds of ancient seas.

It is the overall trace mineral intake they consume that contributes to their long lives plus their diets rich in locally grown fruits and vegetables, which are rich sources of whole-food vitamins C and E.

If we look at centenarian aging studies, we notice several things that long-lived people have in common:

• Increased glutathione reductase and catalase antioxidant activity leading to better physical health and mental function (regenerated by whole-food vitamin C), helping decrease incidence of many chronic diseases associated with aging

• Higher levels of HDL (good) cholesterol—two to three-times what is considered normal, leading to low levels of dementia

- Improved telomere length that slows cellular aging

- Above average growth hormone levels and activity

- Improved cardiovascular function

- Nutrient-rich diet in bioflavonoids (whole-food vitamin C) and antioxidants (including C), vitamins A and E

- Being female

- Genetic factors, including long-lived siblings and healthy variations in the FOXO3A gene, the longevity gene

In recent years, the Okinawans have perfected salt-drying techniques that have given birth to a thriving natural sea-salt industry. These cultures also engage in hard physical labor, eat a comparatively low-calorie diet and walk many miles every day, all of which certainly contribute to their longevity.

WHO now ranks the U.S. an embarrassing 33rd in the world in longevity out of 193 countries. (The Netherlands is number 17.) This U.S. life expectancy statistic has consistently fallen in comparison to other developed countries (in spite of consistent increases in longevity overall) in nearly every decade for the last 50 years. Men's life expectancy in the U.S. is approximately 75 years, women's is 81 years.

If you make it to age 85 in the U.S., there is nearly a 50 percent chance you'll have dementia. Unfortunately dementia is increasing at an alarming rate in the U.S. and there is credible research showing that the use of cholesterol-lowering statin drugs has profound negative effects on the thought process, dramatically increasing memory loss, confusion, depression and cognitive function. The extreme low cholesterol caused by the use of statin drugs is also accelerating mental decline, frailty and early death among elderly people. We need cholesterol for survival—but that's another book.

Our infant mortality has increased in the past decade to 42nd in the developed world from an embarrassing 23rd less than 10 years ago in spite of all our high-risk specialists in the U.S. and our first day death rate is highest in the world. We are the Number 1 worst country—what an embarrassing result!

We could argue about the actual numbers, but seriously, which of these statistics should we be proud of? Our current system is failing miserably due to greed and lack of leadership in implementing significant medical and epidemiologic scientific truths and discoveries in the medical field. It currently takes more than 17 years on the average for a significant health discovery or a scientific confirmation of an error in medical practice to become standard of care. The Calcium Lie is a perfect example. The clock is ticking. It has now been five years since the original publication of this information and it is just now barely becoming part of the consciousness of a few doctors.

That's not a high recommendation considering the technology we have available and the fact that we spend over three times more on our health care than any other developed country in the world, not including the billions spent on supplements. It's interesting to note that the countries with the greatest life expectancies all have diets high in seafood, seaweed and by extrapolation, balanced ionic minerals from the sea.

The Calcium Lie proven in scientific studies

Want another little bit of proof? This study came through just as we were first writing this chapter in the first edition in 2008. It is one of the first of many articles now confirming what I have said in the 2008 edition and again more loudly in this book, and it is even more true today:

An article published in the *British Medical Journal* reported that postmenopausal women who took calcium supplements to maintain bone strength had a dramatically increased risk of a heart attack.

A team of researchers led by Ian Reid, M.D., of the University of Auckland, looked at 1,471 healthy postmenopausal women, average age 74. They gave 732 of the participants a daily calcium supplement of 1,000 milligrams of calcium citrate, while 739 were given a placebo. Participants were followed for five years. The study was originally designed to assess the effect of calcium on bone density and fractures.

During the five-year study period, 31 women on calcium supplements had 45 heart attacks compared to 14 women on placebo who had 19 heart attacks. The same study found that the group that took calcium supplements had almost double the number of heart attacks, strokes and sudden death: 101 events in 69 women vs. 54 events in 42 women not on calcium.

The researchers wrote that the calcium supplements may elevate blood calcium levels and possibly speed calcification in blood vessels, which is known to predict the rates of vascular problems such as heart attack.

Here's some more proof:

Another team of New Zealand-based researchers analyzed 15 large studies (called a meta-analysis) and discovered that people who took 500 mg of calcium supplements a day for one year had a greater risk of heart attacks than those who did not take calcium.

Of 8,151 participants in the studies, 143 people taking calcium supplements had heart attacks, compared to 111 who got placebos.

And here's another really important study that shows that adding vitamin D to calcium probably makes the problem worse:

The journal *Heart* reported on May 24, 2012, an 86 percent increase in heart disease with supplementation with calcium (over 1,100 mg per day) and vitamin D (800 units per day) in 24,000 German people between the ages of 35 and 64, followed for over 11 years.

In another study of 163 "healthy" postmenopausal women ages 57 to 85 presented to the Endocrine Society Annual Meeting in 2012, Christopher Gallagher, M.D., of Creighton University Medical Center, Omaha, NE, revealed that 33 percent of the patients studied at various levels of vitamin D and calcium supplementation experienced significant hypercalcuria (excessively increased urinary calcium levels) increasing the risk of kidney stones. Another 10 percent experienced high levels of calcium in the blood in testing every three months for one year. He concluded, "It is important to monitor blood and urine calcium levels in people who take these supplements on a long-term basis."

I remind the reader that 95 percent of our body's mineral mass is outside the blood, therefore, the most accurate way to determine body mineral levels is hair tissue mineral analysis (HTMA), which specifically assesses the whole body's mineral content. I agree that measurement of these levels is imperative. Ignorance is not bliss when it comes to your mineral levels!

There are more studies listed in the reference section. What is important is that *none* of these studies, *none*, made any attempts to analyze tissue mineral calcium levels or corresponding mineral levels before or after the studies thereby sorting out risk groups; there were very few diet controls, and even then, calcium supplementation has been consistently associated with increased risk of heart disease, vascular disease, heart attack, stroke, kidney stones, plaque, and increased fracture risk or no or minimal protection. This should and eventually will become common knowledge. It is too obvious and too reliable to ignore.

What else do we need to convince the medical profession of the danger of calcium supplementation?

It is time to stop researching this hypothesis that humans need extra calcium in order to have strong bones. It is completely flawed thinking to conclude that calcium supplementation could be uniformly good for us.

We **have to know for sure** our body's mineral levels for our educated doctors to help us know what to eat, how to supplement correctly and, when necessary, which prescription medications to take.

More than 2,400 years ago, Hippocrates summed up today's calcium issue most clearly when he said, "There are, in effect, two things: to know and to believe one knows. To know is science. To believe one knows is ignorance."

POINTS TO REMEMBER

✔ Bones are not made of calcium; they are made of many minerals. Almost all of us get too much calcium since it is contained in many food products and supplements fueled by the flawed thinking that we all need calcium. Those minerals added to your one-a-day "vitamin" supplements are not the answer and may also be harmful.

✔ The minerals we put in our bodies must be water soluble (ionic or salt form and dissolvable) to be absorbed and utilized.

✔ Using refined table salt leaves valuable minerals and trace minerals out of our diet. We need more than iodized salt and calcium for good health and strong bones.

✔ Eating unrefined rock salt from the sea or from land-based salt beds, and taking ionic mineral supplements made from unrefined sea salt will help you restore and maintain your mineral balance.

✔ Our foods don't contain the minerals they once did because of mineral-depleted soil and lack of vine ripening.

✔ Calcium excess causes an increased chance of calcification, concretions, or gravel-like or concrete-like calcium deposits in our arteries (plaque), joints (spurs), eyes (cataracts), brain (shrinkage, dementia), kidneys and gallbladder (stones), and other health issues, including hardening of the arteries, heart disease, dementia, cancer, diabetes, hypothyroidism and hypertension (due to intracellular sodium depletion) to name a few.

CHAPTER 2

The Calcium Myth

THIS CRAZY BELIEF SYSTEM EMBRACING THE BIG LIE about calcium and bones has taken on the fervor of a religion. It's a really dogmatic religion that allows no deviation. The sadly erroneous doctrine says that bones are made of calcium and that calcium builds strong bones. Maybe it's even become a cult.

We're not sure about the origins of this strange and scientifically void idea, but it has somehow made itself part of our collective consciousness. Scientists, nutritionists and medical professionals who are reminded of the basic science that bones are composed of at least 12 essential minerals and many more trace minerals, get some kind of convenient amnesia a day, a week or even a month later, and revert to this strangely insinuated belief system erroneously admonishing: "Get your calcium." Our bones are in fact, the storehouse of all the minerals our bodies need. We know that if we use medications (bisphosphonates like Fosamax) to stop these minerals from leeching out the bones, over time we see an increase of downstream effects, most commonly cardiac muscle or other mineral deficiencies leading to increased risk of atrial fibrillation.

The medical profession, especially radiologists, has quite significantly made the observation that bone mineral density testing (called pDexa) shows that our bone mineral levels decline with age. Helpful hint: This test is *not* called bone calcium density—it's called bone *mineral* density.

What is absurd is that these very intelligent physicians, radiologists and nutritionists fail to recognize that bone density loss is merely a deficiency of minerals in the diet and as nutritional supplements across an entire population. It is not an expected part of aging. To assume otherwise is clearly ignorance or misguided thinking. This observation is too obvious to ignore. It is fact. This decline of bone mineral density is merely an observation of the problem of mineral decline across an entire population. It is not an expected part of aging any more than cancer or heart disease should be expected.

With proper mineral supplementation, declining mineral levels are entirely and completely preventable and most often reversible. This means osteoporosis and related fractures are nearly completely preventable *nutritional* diseases.

We do not need another ten years of calcium research to see the obvious fallacy in the "get your calcium" mantra. We need to replace our minerals daily to keep up with or exceed our losses.

Here's the overarching message of this book: Stop taking calcium and start taking balanced trace minerals. The calcium needed is in the trace minerals. Hair tissue mineral analysis (HTMA) will clarify the specific mineral needs and deficiencies.

I recommend that my patients consume at least three grams of sea salt-derived trace minerals per day. When they do, they consistently have increases in bone mineral density levels over time and their bones stay strong as long as they maintain adequate mineral intake.

With correct supplementation, I have observed increases in bone mineral density of more than 15 percent in less than two years. Remember: Our body tissues are on the average 72 percent water and 28 percent trace minerals.

So I ask my patients, "What are the two most important things we put in our bodies every day?"

The answer is always the same: water (hopefully pure and alkaline), and trace minerals (sea salt-derived low sodium balanced ionic trace minerals).

I now encourage my patients to take trace minerals with every glass of water.

Medical professionals, in particular, often seem to practice a belief system based on everything drug companies say, regardless of significant contradictive observations in other medical studies. They won't budge from these illogical, erroneous and unscientific belief systems. I remind my stubborn colleagues: Belief systems are not scientific fact. Just stick to the facts!

First we have to doubt what we think we know, be epistomocrats and form our practice based on knowledge, not conjecture.

Where did the sacred cow of calcium come from? You're on the right track if you focused on the "sacred cow." Generations of Americans have been programmed through misleading advertising to believe that milk builds strong bones and teeth because of its abundant calcium content. We've known for at least 39 years that this was patently false. The U.S. government even validated the dangers of milk, but old ideas die hard.

In 1974, the Federal Trade Commission forced the California Milk Producers Advisory Board and its advertising agency to stop its "false, misleading and deceptive advertising campaigns" called "Everybody Needs Milk" and "Milk Does a Body Good." Undaunted, the industry launched a new advertising campaign entitled, "Milk Has Something for Everybody." Over time, the advertising buzz morphed to the comparatively innocuous celebrity mustachioed, "Got milk?" campaign intended to trigger our memories of the wonders of milk consumption for "strong" bones.

In fact, all of this is patently false and the research proves it.

Such scientific luminaries as Walter Willett, Ph.D., Chairman of the Department of Nutrition at the Harvard School of Public Health, and T. Colin Campbell, Professor Emeritus of Nutritional Biochemistry at Cornell University, have published research that shows that boosting calcium intake to the currently recommended levels will not prevent fractures. Furthermore, Willett and Campbell suggest excess calcium intake might, in fact, weaken bones and increase fracture risk.

Willett, who co-authored The Nurses' Health Study, one of the largest investigations ever into the risk factors for major chronic diseases in 122,000 women, found that women with the highest calcium consumption from dairy products actually had substantially more fractures than women who consumed less dairy.

We've got a lot more to say about milk and the industry's ongoing efforts to keep us believing The Calcium Lie in future chapters. This problem, unfortunately, has developed long coattails. The Calcium Lie has become so imbedded into our belief systems about healthy food that calcium is now added to many foods, and advertising entices us to buy these "enriched" products. Now we find calcium added to soy milk, orange juice, baby food, cereals, pasta, and—yeeks, imagine this—a genetically modified carrot that contains increased calcium! It's not nice to fool with Mother Nature. Be meticulous in your label reading and avoid the "calcium-enriched" foods unless you know for sure you need them.

We think our readers are smarter than that. We've said it before and we'll say it again: *BONES ARE MADE OF MINERALS*. Yes, one of those minerals is calcium, and yes, calcium is also important, but we create a grave imbalance in the body if we get too much calcium in a misguided effort to build strong bones. Remember: *Calcium hardens concrete and it hardens all sorts of "stuff" in your body, too.*

Bones aren't made of calcium

Here's what bones *are* made of:

• Calcium	• Zinc
• Potassium	• Selenium
• Magnesium	• Boron
• Manganese	• Phosphorus
• Silica	• Sulfur
• Iron	• Chromium
• And traces of 64 other minerals.	

That's what bones are made of, a total of 76 ionizing minerals. Not snakes and snails or puppy dogs' tails and definitely not just calcium. Let's stick with the science. Any sensible person can see that if we want strong bones, we need to keep *all* of these minerals in our bones and in balance. We deplete our stores on a daily basis, and we need to replace them all every day. Replacing just one mineral creates an imbalance that has a cascading effect we'll talk about later in this chapter.

I hear the justifications for calcium supplements virtually every day. They usually go like this: ""I take calcium supplements because I don't get much calcium in my food. Or "I don't drink milk or eat cheese, so I need calcium supplements." Or, worst of all, "I take calcium because my doctor tells me everyone my age is calcium deficient."

These mistakes in thinking continue unabated. We need all the minerals, not just calcium. Think of your complete balanced ionic mineral intake as if your life depends on them. It does.

Is there a way to press the "delete" button and rid our minds once and for all of the misconception about calcium and bones? We'd like to think this is possible, but we know it will take a conscious effort for all of us to change our thought patterns and remember this truth from now on.

Who's winning?

This collective amnesia makes us wonder how many other erroneous misconceptions have been foisted on us by who-knows-who. It is amazing how false advertising used to sell a product can lead to a lie becoming a belief system.

No, we're not conspiracy theorists. We're not the kind of people who see the devil behind every bush. It is strange, however, that these erroneous beliefs are so pervasive and so dogmatically held, not only by the general public, but by doctors, nutritionists and other healthcare professionals who have the tools to know better.

It's also "coincidental" that the big pharmaceutical companies rake in billions upon billions of dollars a year treating the diseases caused by excess calcium in the human body. Big Pharma isn't interested in selling calcium supplements, or at least that's not the major thrust. But pharmaceutical companies are making a fortune from drugs used to treat the diseases that result from calcium excess. We're not making accusations, we're just pointing out the basic facts. Disease is not supposed to be big business.

Here are the facts:

Cardiovascular disease

Heart disease is the Number 1 killer in the United States. In fact, it is the biggest killer in the Western world. The cause of heart disease is not well understood. Common prescription drugs used to prevent and treat hardening of the arteries, literally caused by calcification or excessive amounts of calcium in the arteries (also called calcific plaque—there's a clue), include the statin drugs like Lipitor, Zocor and Crestor. Unfortunately, doctors and patients have been led to believe that cholesterol is the problem. This has been called The Big Fat Lie. In reality, research shows us that people with the lowest cholesterol have the highest death rates from all causes. Higher levels have been proven to be protective against cancer, depression, mental decline and behavioral and addictive disorders.

Just last year, more than 355 million prescriptions were written for these drugs worldwide according to the information from IMS Health, and over 60 percent of all heart attack survivors are taking the drugs in the erroneous belief that statins will prevent another heart attack.

"Thus far there are no documented studies that show any benefit of statin drugs for any woman of any age with any condition. They have not been documented to help people who have not had a previous heart attack of any age or gender," said Dr. Dwight Lundell, author of *The Great Cholesterol Lie.*

Despite all of the so-called "advances" in treatment of heart disease, it remains the Number 1 cause of death in the United States. And the drug companies are raking in over $30 billion *a year* on statin drugs.

A recent study has even shown that Crestor, one of the top-selling statin drugs, was found to have almost no effect in preventing heart attacks during a two-year study, in spite of the billions of dollars spent on the therapy. Another report showed that for every 100 patients on statin drugs, only 2 to 4 heart attacks might be prevented. Side effects of these drugs include memory loss in nearly 70 percent of those who take them, a 250 percent increased risk of developing Alzheimer's disease, nearly 300 percent increase in developing congestive heart disease and liver damage and liver failure. Studies that showed serious risks of liver damage from statins were never published by the drugs' manufacturers.

Additional statin risks are: muscle damage (2.8 times higher with Crestor; at least seven people have died) and kidney failure (found to be 75 times higher with Crestor than with the other statin drugs) and illegally delayed reports of serious adverse side effects by the Crestor manufacturer AstraZeneca, which spent over a billion dollars on marketing this drug alone. And yet the FDA continues to allow the use of these drugs with mere increased warnings to doctors. How about the patients? Who is warning them?

Stephanie Seneff, Ph.D., senior research scientist at MIT, has concluded, "Statin drugs will go down in history as a worse disaster than (synthetic) hormone replacement therapy, Vioxx, and thalidomide combined."

I think she should include The Calcium Lie as an even bigger disaster. The health consequences of these grave errors are staggering especially in view of the easy, cheap and safe alternatives. These include:

- The combination of **soluble fiber** (the Weight Control Formula™ marketed by Life Extension, which has been shown to be equal to Lipitor in lowering bad cholesterol in a head-to-head study);

- Stabilized **rice bran** (featured on Dr. Oz), marketed by Bob's Red Mill and a handful of other licensed companies, is high in whole-food vitamin B3, the real niacin which has no side effects in the whole-food nondrug form and it helps lower bad cholesterol;

- The insulin-resistance reducing product called ChromeMate (chromium polynicotinate) which has a significant effect on lowering triglycerides and LDL cholesterol when taken correctly.

Hypertension

Another case in point: a class of drugs called, interestingly, calcium channel blockers (CCBs). These drugs are meant to combat hypertension or high blood pressure by blocking calcium's role in contracting muscles in the heart and arteries and relaxing muscles, thus directly lowering blood pressure. Of course, if there were no excess calcium in the body in the first place, these drugs might not be necessary. If there is a calcium excess and hypertension, this medication class may be even more effective or medically necessary.

For nearly eight years now, we have known that CCBs are dangerous. We've known it since a paper was presented at the European Cardiology Society blaming the calcium channel blockers for causing 85,000 avoidable heart attacks and cases of heart failure *each year.* If the excess calcium doesn't get into the cells or intracellular spaces, it gets deposited in the arteries. But these drugs remain among the most popular drugs for heart disease, with 92 million prescriptions filled for the drugs in the U.S. alone in 2009. And they net the drug companies at least $4.5 billion a year from American sales alone (2011 figures, IMS Health).

Statins and CCBs are just two of an enormous number of prescription drugs used to treat the effects of excessive amounts of calcium in the arteries. They are frequently prescribed without even knowing if excess calcium is really the problem, although it usually is. Similarly, the common thought in management of hypertension is sodium restriction. This is the wrong treatment if the patient already is severely sodium depleted intracellularly. We have to know for sure the mineral content of our bodies before we can validate any and all healthcare recommendations, including diet and drugs.

The correct treatment for all hypertension depends on knowing the intracellular levels of these most important minerals. Without knowing for certain, doctors are merely guessing and these professionals who pride themselves on a "scientific approach" are frequently guessing wrong.

You can extrapolate the numbers for yourself. The pharmaceutical profits are mind-boggling. And if they just treat the symptoms, they don't get you better and they may make you worse.

You've probably already noticed that we keep repeating certain phrases, like "Calcium hardens concrete, not bones" and "We have to know for sure."

We're not absentminded. It's intentional. We want to repeat these concepts often to help undo the brainwashing we've all suffered at the hands of Big Pharma, the dairy industry and the medical community. Such ideas warrant frequent repetition because they are new to most of us and vitally important to our health.

Based on my experience, it appears that at least 90 percent of all hypertension is being treated incorrectly.

When we say, "We need to know for sure," I'm referring to hair tissue mineral analysis (HTMA). You'll hear lots more about this important test in the coming chapters, but for now it's important to know that I recommend it for all patients, especially in those with hypertension.

In more than 12 years of experience with these concepts, treating nearly 2000 patients, and with worldwide sampling, I know that 90 percent of the world's population is severely sodium deficient. You'll learn later why sodium deficiency is closely linked to most hypertension.

Every treatment and every medication recommendation should be based on *knowing* the exact mineral imbalance and deficiencies you are treating. The goal of every correct treatment should be to correct the problem, not just to treat the symptoms.

Obesity

Yes, you read it right. Excess calcium in the human body leads to most obesity. Think of a body starved for minerals and the other nutrients that those minerals allow your body to absorb and use. This may seem like a stretch of logic, but we assure you, an overweight body is literally starving for the nutrients (especially minerals) it needs, so it puts out signals that create cravings in an attempt to get you to eat *something* that will nourish it.

Now we know most of us don't get cravings for spinach or salmon. This desperate attempt to find nutritional nourishment causes us to crave sugary, salty and fatty foods that are so destructive to our health. Worst of all, it sets up a vicious cycle of cravings. The failure to satisfy those cravings leads to increasingly urgent signals that our brains misinterpret and this stimulates unhealthy eating. Sometimes these cravings can also lead to other compulsive and addictive behaviors.

Now think of the diet industry. We're talking about over-the-counter diet drugs, the ubiquitous ads that invade our airwaves constantly urging us to buy diet plans and supplements with calcium added. Of course, there are also the prescription drugs and surgeries that promise to help us lose weight and keep it off. All that comes at a very high cost, and I'm not just talking about your pocketbook.

Interestingly, the average diet-drink consumer, thinking that avoiding sugar will help control weight, actually increases the risk of obesity (and type 2 diabetes) for every can of diet soft drink consumed, substantially more than those who drink regular sugared soft drinks. For example, drinking one to two cans of diet soft drinks a day increases your risk of obesity by 54.5 percent as opposed to the increased risk of a comparatively small 32.8 percent if you drink one to two cans of sugared soft drinks daily. Neither is good, but you can see the difference. The probable cause is that artificial sweeteners in diet soft drinks stimulate appetite and increase insulin resistance.

These numbers from a University of Texas study were presented to the American Diabetes Association (ADA) in 2005. Yet there has not been an ADA statement to date condemning the widespread use of diet soft drinks by diabetics. So who gains here? We think you're getting the picture.

Fatty liver, a common problem in obese people, is accelerated when they are on statin drugs, which poison the liver's ability to metabolize fructose found in soft drinks. This may explain the increased risk of liver failure with statin drugs.

Jenny Craig, just one popular prepared-foods diet plan, reported sales of over $400 million in 2006. The company was purchased by Nestle for $600 million in 2006. The diet business as a whole reportedly generates about $50 billion a year in income just for over-the counter food plans.

That number doesn't even begin to touch the proceeds of prescription diet drugs and surgeries, or the multitudinous and well-documented cost of health conditions related to obesity. Nor does it count for the many nutritional supplements that claim to aid in weight loss.

Once again, we need to treat the underlying causes of obesity, that is insulin resistance, hypothyroidism (including type 2 "resistance" to the thyroid hormone), and mineral imbalances that also affect metabolic rate. Not treating the underlying causes will cause successful dieters to regain weight and get back on the weight roller coaster.

Type 2 diabetes

Whoa! This is a big bonanza for Big Pharma. Not only do the drugs to treat diabetes bring in big bucks, there are all those drugs used to treat the heart disease, obesity, kidney and eye diseases that almost inevitably accompany diabetes, just to name a few.

We're just touching the tip of the iceberg here, but just consider this: 2006 sales of a newer class of drugs for treating type 2 diabetes called glitazones (brand names Avandia and Actos) were well over $6 billion, despite studies that go back as far as 1999 suggesting that these drugs increase the risk of heart attack in an already heart-attack prone diabetic population. Avandia has also been linked to bladder cancer.

There are several more drugs commonly used to treat type 2 diabetes, all of them quite profitable for their manufacturers. In their annual reports, drug manufacturers have crowed about the double-digit increase in sales over the past few years. Obviously, there is a lot more money to be made in the treatment of diabetes than in the prevention of the disease.

Treating and preventing type 2 diabetes can be simpler, safer, cheaper and almost completely effective. Through nutrition and correct supplementation, I have successfully eliminated type 2 diabetes in over 100 adult patients and completely eliminated gestational diabetes in nearly 100 percent of my pregnant patients.

Brain function

In general, excess calcium causes brain cells to stop working. Brain cells that govern memory normally have an approximate outside/inside calcium concentration ratio of 1,000:1. This means that even a tiny influx of calcium into the brain cells will cause huge functional consequences.

Calcium excess has been linked to impairment of brain function that can result in rapid brain aging, brain shrinkage, cell death and increased risk of dementia and Alzheimer's disease. Quincy Bioscience has developed a supplement called Prevagen, a jellyfish-derived protein, identical to the protein in humans that specifically helps keep calcium from going into the brain. Its use has been shown to reduce brain cell death by up to 50 percent. If you are over the age of 50 and in the 90 percent of people with HTMA results showing high intracellular calcium levels, supplementing with this product could be very important in protecting your brain from the calcium excess and dementia at least until the calcium excess resolves.

Joe R's Story

Joe R was a healthy middle-aged man who exercised regularly, ate fairly healthy food and was at his ideal body weight. He thought he was in great shape. Unfortunately, he had become somewhat of a diet soft drink addict in the past few years, drinking five or six cans of liquid death a day.

Now, Joe knew that diabetes ran in his family. His father, an aunt and a sister had diabetes, but he thought it would never happen to him. After all, he told me, he watched his diet and exercised, so he was safe. Right? Wrong. When Joe was scheduled for routine knee surgery back in 1997, pre-operative blood tests showed he had an elevated fasting blood sugar of 128. That's enough to diagnose insulin resistance and many doctors consider it means the patient has full-blown type 2 diabetes.

Within 10 months, Joe was showing all the classic signs of type 2 diabetes. He had lost 15 to 20 pounds without trying and he wasn't happy about it. He was running to the bathroom 15 times a day, the result of a raging thirst that he never seemed to be able to quench. Simple finger-stick blood tests showed his fasting blood sugar levels were in the danger zone at 150–200 and 250–350 after eating.

We did a hair tissue mineral analysis (HTMA) and the results were surprising: Joe had very low chromium levels, which I attributed to his diet soft drink obsession. We now know that NutraSweet (aspartame) in soft drinks depletes chromium, among other things.

I started Joe on a variety of simple supplements and minerals, including mealtime doses of ChromeMate™, a specialized form of chromium, sometimes referred to as GTF Chromium, that would help replace the depleted chromium stores, improve his ability to process sugars and his body's ability to use insulin.

Joe's results were really impressive: Within two weeks all his blood sugars were within the normal range.

He remained on the supplement regimen for the next year and his blood sugars remained normal.

I have followed Joe for more than 15 years. He now takes a dramatically reduced number of supplements and his daily minerals to keep his blood sugars at normal levels. We know, because we make sure Joe gets his glucose and insulin tested every three months. His most recent fasting glucose was 99—well within the normal range. I consider that a cure for a disease that is supposedly incurable. In my experience, type 2 diabetes is nearly always curable or reversible, if it's caught early enough. Joe's story and those of over 100 other patients I've treated with this program are all the confirmation I need.

Hypothyroidism

One drug manufacturer boasted that more than 6 million people around the world use its thyroid hormones and another reported 2005 sales of a comparatively paltry $500 million. We will discuss the role of calcium in the development of type 2 hypothyroidism (thyroid hormone resistance) in detail in Chapter 5, but for now, we'll tell you that excess calcium causes metabolic failures and nowhere is this more apparent than in thyroid malfunction. In my practice, nearly 95 percent of women over the age of 40 exhibit signs of type 2 hypothyroidism, which I also call thyroid hormone resistance. It's not coincidental that virtually every single one of them has excess intracellular calcium as determined by their HTMA.

After many years of studying, networking with other health professionals and applying HTMA results to the mix, my understanding of this disease has greatly increased. I have concluded that there are at least five different types of hypothyroidism, easily distinguishable, specifically treatable, and at least four of the types may be reversible with the correct treatments.

Osteoarthritis, kidney stones and gallstones

All of these conditions are the result of excess calcium being dumped in the intercellular spaces in joints, and into the kidneys and the gall bladder. Arthritis drugs alone brought in $18 billion in worldwide sales in 2004. Of those, the controversial COX-2 inhibitors like Celebrex and Vioxx brought in close to $7 billion. Fortunately, Vioxx was withdrawn from the market that year after studies showed it dramatically increased the risk of heart attack and stroke. Celebrex and its look-alike, Bextra, remain available with healthy sales, and safety questions are still pending.

Several studies have now shown that calcium supplementation for the "prevention" of or "treatment" of osteoporosis increases the risk of kidney stones.

Migraines

Sales from just one popular migraine drug, Imitrex (sumatriptan succinate), and a related drug, called Imigran, totaled $1.315 billion in 2006. Imitrex's patent expired in 2009, but its manufacturer introduced and received FDA approval for a "new and improved" version called Treximet with added naproxen (Aleve—an over-the-counter anti-inflammatory). Generic forms of Imitrex are now available for less than $5 a dose compared to $25 or more for Treximet. We will explain in more detail the connection between calcium excess and neurotransmitter deficiencies, in this case serotonin, in Chapter 4.

We think we've gone far enough with these examples to let you know who has the most to gain from our health woes. Yes, we know it sounds cynical and we hope and pray we are wrong, but the circumstantial evidence is certainly damning.

The Calcium Cascade

Excess calcium in the human body begins a cascade of negative effects that have enormous adverse consequences to our health. This process cannot be diagnosed with standard blood tests. It requires a reliable, competent lab to conduct a hair tissue mineral analysis (HTMA) on a correctly collected hair sample you provide. I recommend Trace Elements Inc., the only lab with the correct ratios and databases. You can find information about them in the resources section and through my website, www.calciumlie.com.

Warning: Here comes some more basic biochemistry or human physiology. We'll try to keep it as simple and painless as possible.

If you have excess or relative calcium excess in your body

THAT LEADS TO

Calcium seeking and needing more magnesium to try to keep your body's
calcium and magnesium in balance

THAT LEADS TO

A relative magnesium deficiency in proportion to calcium that leads to
increased muscle tension, and nerve endings firing erratically
and other "electrical" malfunctions in your body;

AND

In its need for more magnesium, your body has to suppress adrenal function
in order to retain more magnesium to compensate for the high calcium.
This adrenal suppression causes a continuous loss of sodium
and potassium in your urine as well as immune compromise
from the adrenal suppression.

THIS LEADS TO

A continual depletion of the sodium and potassium that are stored
inside the trillions of cells in your body;

THAT LEADS TO

A loss of the sodium and chloride you need to produce the stomach acid
you need to digest protein;

AND

This increases the incidences of heartburn and other digestive disorders, and the use of prescription drugs that have further destructive effects and impede digestion;

AND

Your body gradually loses its ability to digest protein and absorb the essential amino acids that are the building blocks of protein and neurotransmitters.

ALSO

The sodium depletion leads to a failure of membrane electrical potential and ion exchanges necessary for cellular function, the mechanism by which our bodies get essential amino acids and glucose into all our cells, except fat cells which keep absorbing glucose without sodium while the rest of our bodies cells are starving.

FURTHERMORE

Intracellular potassium levels decline dramatically and this leads to increasing degrees of thyroid hormone resistance (type 2 hypothyroidism), with all the symptoms of hypothyroidism and slowed metabolism with what are thought to be normal blood tests. Correct diagnosis requires blood tests, HTMA, basal body temperatures and total and reverse T3 ratio.

SO

All cells (except fat cells) become starved for glucose and amino acids,

RESULTING IN

Increased cravings for glucose and increased food intake. This loss of minerals also leads to more food cravings

AND

Intracellular deficiencies of sodium, potassium and essential amino acids, and more cravings.

THE END RESULT IS

Multiple metabolic malfunctions, including, obesity, heart disease, type 2 hypothyroidism, type 2 diabetes, anxiety, migraines, depression, dementia, hypertension
and the list goes on and on!

We'll discuss all of the implications of the calcium cascade and sodium/potassium membrane potential electrical failure in the coming chapters. For now, if all of this biochemistry threatens to overwhelm you, you need to know that excess calcium in your system can be an underlying factor in a host of deadly health problems.

Too much calcium messes up your entire physiology. Now that doesn't mean you don't need some calcium. You do. We all need some calcium, but 95 percent of us don't need anywhere near the amount of calcium we get. Our calcium intake must be in correct proportions to the intake of all the other minerals our bodies need. We need balanced trace minerals, not just calcium.

It doesn't matter what kind of calcium supplement you take or the hype about so-called "super" forms of calcium like coral calcium. Calcium is calcium and you remember what calcium does, right? Calcium hardens concrete.

Remember: Bones are made of minerals. We keep repeating this mantra to help you break the reflexive adherence to The Calcium Lie.

I estimate that we need at least 3,000 milligrams of sea salt–derived trace minerals per day and this is probably conservative. This assumes that you have no deficiencies, no imbalances and no excess calcium, and you are in great physiologic health already and not pregnant. In more than 12 years of analyzing mineral statuses and treating nearly 2,000 patients, I have seen only one patient who had no deficiencies at all, and his imbalances were minimal. This is a rare patient. We all need to know our tissue mineral levels and ratios to meaningfully improve our health.

How do you know if you have excess calcium?

How can you tell if you have too much calcium in your system? The answer is simple, but the correction process may not be as simple.

First, you need a test called a hair tissue mineral analysis (HTMA). All you'll need to do is clip a small amount of new growth of undyed clean hair, each piece about $1/2$ to $3/4$ inches long from an average of three spots on your head nearest to the scalp and send it to your doctor. I recommend that you find a physician trained in this area who is already using a TEI (Trace Elements Inc.) lab, the only lab I feel is completely competent

From Dr. Thompson

What does this all mean?

Over the past 12 years of ordering comprehensive tissue mineral analyses, my experience has shown that more than 90 percent of my patients have calcium excess or relative calcium excesses, ranging from significant to extreme.

I can only relate this to my medical practice. I have found that this is a fairly typical populace issue worldwide as I consult with patients from various countries and various states (except New York where HTMA is prohibited by the medical board due to ignorance).

This calcium excess seems to be the highest in the younger generations and in dairy consumers. It is significantly associated with nearly all obesity. The parents and grandparents typically also have both the calcium excess and serious mineral deficiencies. These results are based on tissue mineral analysis tests conducted by Trace Elements, Inc. (TEI) in Addison, Texas, whose director, Dr. David Watts, PhD, D.C., FACEP, has conducted more than 1,000,000 tissue mineral profiles over the past 23 years. This company has developed an impressive database showing the relationships between minerals, vitamins, the human metabolism and a wide variety of disease processes. Dr. Watts is one of the few medical professionals who truly understands the dangers of calcium excess and mineral imbalances. I don't have any financial interest in his company, but I wish I did!

You and your doctor must know for sure what mineral imbalances you have and HTMA is the only way you can truly know for sure.

Forgive me. I'm passionate about this. The entire developed world is on the brink of a health crisis that we cannot afford. Sadly, this will extend to the next generation and the one after that with increasing health consequences at earlier ages, if we don't do something to reverse it now.

to do a proper analysis. To find such doctors, visit our website, www. calciumlie.com, A4M.org and/or ACAM.org. Hopefully the use of this test will become common in all medical practices after this book is released.

Your results will give you important information about your intracellular levels of 36 minerals, including calcium, magnesium, sodium and potassium. You'll also get information about the most important ratios of minerals that are critical to your entire metabolism, levels of important trace minerals and levels of toxic minerals. The report includes specific information for each individual on the meaning of the results and recommends specific dietary ways to address imbalances. I always individualize the results and often make specific additional nutritional recommendations based on my experience with the test and nutritional awareness.

The tissue mineral analysis test at this lab is only available through a qualified healthcare provider, so you'll need a good doctor or healthcare provider to guide you through interpreting the test results and developing a treatment regimen. That's the hard part. There simply aren't many doctors who are aware of The Calcium Lie, and fewer yet who have any idea what to do about it.

Your insurance company may resist paying for it; however, TEI is a government-certified lab. I have had patients challenge the nonpayment, and I'm finding that an increasing percentage of insurance companies are covering the test. It's an investment in your health that is well worth the cost. It may be the most important medical health test you will have in your lifetime.

Blood tests are not as accurate as the HTMA in determining our body's mineral levels because the calcium levels outside the cells or in the blood as well as concentrations of many other essential mineral levels can differ greatly from those inside the cells. By analyzing new hair growth we get a picture of the mineral levels inside of the cells of our largest organ, the skin; we can thereby get an accurate picture of the mineral profile of the inside of the cells of the entire body.

You might begin your search by looking at our website, www.calcium lie.com where we hope to someday have a list of doctors who can submit and analyze and interpret your HTMA results. A doctor who is a member of one of these professional societies that are dedicated to open thought processes in integrative medicine may be helpful:

- The American College for Advancement in Medicine, an association of integrative health practitioners: www.acam.org, phone: 949-309-3520.

- The American Academy of Anti-Aging Medicine (A4M), which has doctors worldwide who are dedicated to preventive health: www.world health.net, phone: 773-528-1000.

I hope the folks at these wonderful organizations will be able to help you find the right doctor.

If not, you'll have to educate your own doctor. Be prepared. This unfortunately is likely to be a long and difficult process. You can start by providing a copy of this book and perhaps a copy of Chapter 10 entitled "Doctor to Doctor: An Impassioned Plea." You can also keep yourself and your doctor up to date by regularly visiting our website: www.calcium lie.com. We'll be posting new information there frequently.

Our challenge to other physicians is that they should care more about their patients. They don't really have to know everything; they just have to be willing to listen to their patients and be open to changing their ingrained thought and learning processes. I often say to my colleagues, "Patients do not care about how much you know, they care about how much you care." It is logical to conclude that a caring physician will want to know and learn more, and not be completely stuck in old and erroneous beliefs.

In addition to getting your HTMA and following the dietary instructions you'll find in Chapter 9, you'll need to begin taking mineral supplements right away. I always recommend that my patients immediately begin taking a high quality ionic mineral supplement made by Trace Mineral Research or Research Minerals, Inc. They have several forms. Please use only the one with my name on the label. I do not endorse the others.

You must know your mineral analysis results to be sure you get the correct supplement. However, either of these is better than none. I recommend taking at least six of the mineral tablets per day (3,000 mg) or about two teaspoons of the liquid trace minerals. The liquid tastes nasty, so dilute it slightly into about one to two ounces of water and "chug" it.

These supplements do contain calcium and that's OK, because calcium naturally occurs in sea salt in the right proportions. The supplements (and unrefined sea salt) all contain calcium in the perfect proportion with other minerals so it works for you rather than against you. You may also need some other whole-food supplements and dietary changes, which we'll address in Chapter 9.

POINTS TO REMEMBER

✔ Bones are not made of calcium. They are made of a dozen or more minerals, all of which are essential to bone strength.

✔ Calcium supplements, milk and dietary calcium do not produce strong bones. Minerals in proper balance produce strong bones. Osteoporosis is a loss of minerals, not just calcium, from the bones.

✔ Remember the Calcium Cascade in which excess calcium starts causing adrenal suppression in order for the body to retain magnesium to compensate. This leads to sodium and potassium loss from our cells and then out through the urine and an increased proportion of calcium in our cells. Adrenal suppression and adrenal hormone resistance results, with continuous loss of sodium, which eventually shuts down protein digestion and glucose and amino acid transport into cells, and potassium loss, with the relative calcium increase in our cells which leads to type 2 Hypothyroidism (thyroid hormone resistance), and this creates a host of metabolic problems and failures ranging from heart disease, diabetes and obesity to anxiety, migraines, depression, dementia and more.

✔ Calcium excess may be toxic to the brain and significantly contributes to dementia and Alzheimer's disease.

✔ Get a reliable hair tissue mineral analysis (HTMA) available through www.calciumlie.com to determine your personal calcium and other essential mineral, trace mineral and toxic mineral levels, and information about important ratios of these essential minerals that affect our health and metabolism.

✔ Take a high quality ionic trace minerals supplement made from unrefined sea salt minus some of the sodium. Adjust your diet as necessary to accommodate your new correct calcium lifestyle and increased mineral intake. Cooking with the many variations of sea salt is very interesting and significantly increases flavor.

CHAPTER 3

Osteoporosis, Osteoarthritis and Calcium

S O NOW YOU'VE GOT IT. Your bones are not made of calcium, so it stands to reason that osteoporosis, osteopenia and general brittle bones are not caused by a lack of calcium. Nor can you strengthen your bones by taking calcium supplements, drinking lots of milk or eating loads of dairy products and calcium-rich and calcium-fortified foods, no matter what you doctor might tell you.

In fact, you may remember from Chapter 2 that the Harvard and Cornell research on 122,000 women who participated in the Nurses' Health Study showed those who drank the most milk had the highest fracture rates. You now have the knowledge to understand why this is so.

What really causes osteoporosis? If you've read Chapters 1 and 2 carefully, you can probably guess the answer: Osteoporosis is caused by mineral deficiency. It's a loss of the bone structure, the superstructure of your body, because your body doesn't have adequate supplies of *all* the minerals it needs to build strong bones or it has too much of one of those minerals: calcium.

Let's take a little closer look at what happens when we become mineral deficient. Bones are the storehouses of minerals for the entire body, so when any of your trillions of bodily processes is in need of a particular mineral, it goes to the bones for what it needs. Think of your bones as a savings account for minerals. The earlier you make deposits (ideally between puberty and age 30), the stronger your bones will be throughout your life. If the needed mineral isn't there, your body may substitute a similar one, but not without consequences.

Thompson-Döbereiner Mineral Substitution Hypothesis
(my theory and from my personal experience)

Bear with me; this is complex but extremely important new biochemistry:

I am convinced that this process occurs according to the principle of Döbereiner's triads first described in 1817 and possibly with some influences according to the law of octaves, which treats the elements as a repeating scale of musical notes where the note repeats every eight steps.

A simple explanation is that certain elements of the periodic table have very similar biochemical properties. Before the periodic table of elements was completed as the elements were being discovered, it was predicted that certain elements existed based on these minute differences. These similar properties and the principle of mineral substitution have been seen in HTMA results for years, repeatedly observed and associated with specific disease pathologies. Yet the physiology of such examples has had little or no research that I am aware of. According to this "Thompson-Döbereiner Theory," actually knowing the mineral concentrations and ratios of elements in human cells, these substitution principles can be more clearly understood, leading to a new understanding of human disease.

So getting back to the basics, you're right, osteoporosis is not a deficiency of calcium; it's a deficiency of minerals. But osteoporosis is not just a deficiency of minerals in the bones, it's a deficiency of minerals in *the entire body.*

From nearly 2,000 patients I've treated over the past 13 years and from the database of over 1,000,000 HTMA (hair tissue mineral analyses) conducted by Dr. David Watts over the past 25 years, I can say without reservation that more than 95 percent of us are mineral deficient and more than 90 percent of us have too much intracellular calcium. I have convincing evidence that this is a worldwide problem.

And the mineral deficiency problem is getting worse. We'll go into the details in Chapter 6 when we talk about pregnancy and childbirth, but here's what you need to know: A baby will be born with a near exact fingerprint of its mother's mineral status, so if the mother's mineral status is poor, the baby's will be, too. As time goes on, everyone's mineral status typically declines, so the picture for each succeeding generation is worse, especially when we consider the severe deficiencies of these essential minerals and other nutrients in our food. These shortfalls in our environment, our nutrition and in our nutritional lifestyle add up to declining mineral status throughout our lives. This is completely preventable and treatable with proper mineral supplementation. I have concluded that it is impossible to eat to be healthy. In our world today, the quality of our health depends on the accuracy and quality of our diet and supplementation.

What is disturbing is that the medical profession and nutritionists have observed this mineral decline with aging for many years and concluded that this is part of the "normal aging" process. They actually consider an expected decline in mineral levels as we age as "normal" as seen on bone density testing results called pDEXA scores.

This is preposterous. It is a complete denial of the nutritional problem we face across our entire worldwide populations caused by a total lack of adequate mineral nutrients in our food and soil and lack of appropriate supplementation of balanced sea salt-derived trace minerals. The misguided fear of developing high blood pressure from sodium has also been a deterrent to the use of sea salt, depriving us all of essential nutrition and minerals. The use of refined "table salt" has also compounded the problem. I consider table salt the nutritional equivalent of white bread: useless and possibly harmful.

This "expected" decline in mineral levels as we age is merely the documentation of the nutritional problem. It is not necessary and definitely not normal and should never be tolerated.

Adequate trace mineral supplementation is simply essential to healthy bones and overall health. My patients routinely experience meaningful increases in bone density, sometimes 15 percent or more in less than two years with good compliance in taking their trace mineral supplements. The health of our bones should only be compared to healthy minerally dense bone. To recognize and treat mineral deficiency with calcium and vitamin D is equally absurd thinking and will never be accurate science. We must abandon this false hypothesis and move on with accurate balanced ionic trace mineral replacement.

When I see a teenager's HTMA these days, I find as much as 85 percent depletion in the total body mineral content in almost every single case. The excess of calcium that is causing the numerous other imbalances and metabolic failures is the same or worse in young people who should be strong and vibrant, yet they are already at high risk for serious health problem because of mineral imbalances.

When I see the severe levels of mineral depletions in the elderly, it is a tragedy. The average senior's mineral levels are between 5 and 15 percent of normal, with 90 percent having high intracellular calcium and desperately low intracellular sodium and potassium levels of between 7.5 and 15 percent of normal. (See the "Calcium Cascade" in this book to understand the simple physiology that explains this.)

Without enough minerals in the right proportions, your body can't make enough of the hydroxyapatite crystals that make up bone matrix and build bone strength. Without adequate minerals, bones are weakened, more prone to injury and unable to supply the rest of the body with minerals needed for other functions. Without the real vitamin C, the connective tissue around bone is also weakened.

Bone density tests (pDEXA or DEXA scan)

These are diagnostic tests for osteoporosis recommended by nearly every doctor for women over 50. However, the American College of Obstetrics and Gynecology (ACOG) has suggested waiting until age 65, unless specific risk factors are identified. This is too late!

We already know that almost everyone's body mineral levels are severely depleted. Research shows us that a significant percentage of the postmenopausal bone mineral loss occurs in the first two years after menopause.

Unfortunately, these bone mineral density test results are standardized to compare the bone mineral density to others our own age rather than comparing us to a healthy bone density. As our collective bone density worsens, the averages are lower. This is the misguided "expected" decline described above, but for some reason, this is acceptable to most doctors. T-scores may actually improve with age when there is no actual increase in bone density, falsely suggesting that people are improving if they just stay at the same level of mineral deficiency. This is blindness to the problem, which is mineral deficiency across the entire aging population.

Since we know that virtually everyone is mineral deficient, we really should be comparing ourselves to the bones of a healthy 20-year-old. Even at that, we really don't know what "normal" levels should be, based upon our current civilization's nutritional and mineral deficits. TEI has done extensive research into these levels based on studies on ancient civilizations. I call these true normal levels. They are what we should strive to achieve if we want to improve our health and eliminate osteoporosis from our societies.

Finally, bone mineral density is not called bone calcium density. Remember, bone mineral density is just another way to get a measurement of total body mineral levels. However, it is less specific and less accurate than tissue mineral levels. HTMA measures specific mineral levels and determines which ones are missing and presents ratios that indicate which ones are out of balance. This is information we must have in order to make correct nutritional and medical therapeutic choices.

Forgive us a brief aside here: Bones and teeth are composed of the same minerals, so the health of your teeth can be a direct indicator of your bone status.

The National Osteoporosis Foundation (NOF) tells us that 44 million Americans have compromised bone density (either osteoporosis or osteopenia, low bone density that often leads to fractures). By 2020, half of all Americans over 50 are expected to have low bone density. Now we know the NOF people mean well when they tell you to take calcium and "vitamin" D hormone to keep your bones strong. But they're wrong. Dead wrong.

The statistics substantiate the mineral decline and the fact that no matter how much calcium we take, it doesn't make our bones stronger. Bones are made of minerals and calcium is only one mineral. Calcium actually makes bones weaker because it exaggerates our mineral imbalances and deficiencies. Calcium excess causes other essential minerals, especially potassium and sodium, to be lost or excreted in the urine.

And by the way, if you think osteoporosis and osteopenia are diseases of elderly women, think again. True, more than 55 percent of *all people* over the age of 50 have some form of bone deterioration, but 20 percent of those sufferers are men. Today, over 2 million men have been diagnosed with osteoporosis and 12 million are at risk. Anyone can get it, and more and more of us are getting it every day.

If you stop putting extra calcium in your body and replace all the lost minerals instead, the downstream effects of calcium excess will ease over time and you'll find yourself coming back into balance. Knowing your levels and imbalances can make a substantial difference in your health and even change the potential for illness now and in the future. Dietary changes and supplement recommendations must be guided by your HTMA results. To treat patients or make diet or supplement recommendations without this critical information is just plain misguided. If you replace these trace minerals faithfully over time and restore balance, you'll almost always get improvement in current health problems and this replacement and balancing may also prevent many new ones from developing. Nutritional guidance and reliable supplementation recommendations by a healthcare practitioner well instructed in The Calcium Lie, HTMA use, and in nutritional and supplement management based on this information are essential to being truly healthy.

I continually emphasize to my patients how many minerals they need because many of these essential nutrients cannot be found in today's food supply. A minimum of five or six tablets of sea-salt-derived minerals daily (about 3 grams), or two teaspoons of liquid ionic sea-salt-derived trace minerals will just replace what you lose every day, provided you are not pregnant, when you need much more. But those six tablets won't get you ahead of the deficiency. Depending on the results of the HTMA, most of my patients need 9 to 15 tablets a day, at least for several months and sometimes for several years, to correct mineral deficiencies and begin to bring their mineral levels back to normal.

The two most important things we put into our bodies every day are water and trace minerals. Our bodies are on the average 72 percent water and 28 percent minerals.

So, the correct answer to almost all of my teaching questions is "minerals." For example, "Osteoporosis is a loss of what from the bones?" Please do not say calcium, ever again.

Based on this simple truth, we all should be taking trace minerals with every glass of water. I have been working on my tissue mineral levels for over 15 years and they keep improving yearly. However, I still have a way to go. These corrections are a process, a reliable recipe for health improvement, not a destination. When I began taking trace minerals with every glass of water, after only one year, I had the largest improvement in my tissue mineral level I had seen in 12 years. I strongly encourage this if deficiency exists. *We have to know* our HTMA results and eat and supplement correctly to truly improve our health.

Pharmaceuticals for osteoporosis

There is a class of pharmaceuticals for osteoporosis called bisphosphonates. Sold under brand names like Fosamax, Boniva, Actonel and Reclast, these drugs harden bones and prevent further bone deterioration and fractures in people with osteoporosis by slowing the natural resorption and remodeling process, making the bones super hard.

By doing this, the mineral storehouse gets shut down and more mineral imbalances and deficiencies occur in all the cells of the body, making the mineral bank account continuously overdrawn, with far-reaching consequences, as you'll see in the coming chapters. Cellular mineral depletion is actually accelerated if you are using bisphosphonates and if balanced ionic trace minerals are not being adequately replaced daily.

There is another price to pay for these artificially "strengthened" bones. There have been no good long-term studies on bisphosphonates, but some experts theorize that over time, these superhardened bones may shatter if they are fractured, just like a piece of hardened plastic smashed with a hammer.

There have been studies that show bisphosphonates can cause a condition called aseptic bone necrosis, in which the blood supply to the bone is interrupted and the bone quite literally dies.

There are documented cases where bone necrosis has killed the bone in the jaw, resulting in teeth falling out. Hyperbaric oxygen treatment may be the only hope for these patients to save their teeth. It's not a pretty picture.

Using bisphosphonates will slow bone loss in patients with osteoporosis and osteopenia, but these drugs continually rob the rest of the body's cells of their mineral storehouse, so your cells' mineral needs are continually unmet.

In the long term, bisphosphonates may contribute to a vicious cycle of other serious health problems, most significantly, atrial fibrillation.

Bisphosphonates have been shown to be associated with increased rates of atrial fibrillation, a condition in which the heart beats inefficiently and irregularly, raising the risk of blood clots and strokes.

These anti-osteoporotic drugs may be a last resort among people who are already severely compromised in terms of their bone structure, since even supplementation with balanced sea salt-derived ionic minerals alone may not restore this much lost bone fast enough without stopping the loss. I do prescribe them on occasion because of the critical degree of the bone loss in some patients, and there seems to be no better alternative. I always simultaneously recommend, however, as much mineral supplementation as possible along with dietary changes and supplements, guided by the hair tissue mineral analysis results. I use this medication group for the shortest amount of time possible and quickly taper doses over time as pDEXA scores improve with copious trace mineral supplementation and diet changes and supplements guided by the actual HTMA results.

Given all these potential problems, prevention is clearly the best route to take. The more physically active you are early in life (in early teens and even before), the lower your risk of osteoporosis. The more weight-bearing exercise you do, at any stage in life, the lower your risk. This means walking, running, cross-country skiing, tennis, soccer and any of a wide number of activities that keep you on your feet. Recent research shows that it is never too late to start.

Most conventional doctors will want to add calcium to the bisphosphonates and recommend vitamin D supplements as well. We repeat: Don't go there without knowing! The chances that you need supplemental calcium are extremely small, and it is more likely that calcium is going to add to your mineral imbalances and resulting health risks. Excess vitamin D hormone supplements are not advisable if there is already a calcium excess and specifically a calcium/magnesium imbalance. Vitamin D is not a vitamin. It's a hormone because it meets all the classic definitions of a hormone. More is not necessarily better for any hormone regardless of many claims. Our bodies naturally stop producing D hormone when the levels are adequate, even with continued sun exposure.

I routinely correct the deficiency of the vitamin D hormone (it's really not a vitamin) keeping the levels in between 35–60 ng/mL, and never above 60, especially if there is an intracellular calcium excess reported by HTMA testing. This is especially important in patients who already have an intracellular calcium excess. This was a logical compromise to the health risks associated with D deficiency and the calcium excess problems as we have expressed them when we wrote the first book.

After over five years of follow-up with this recommendation, I can conclusively state that this recommendation was correct. Correcting the deficiency of the D hormone has not had negative effects on tissue calcium levels in any follow-up studies on HTMA comparison results in any of my patients unless calcium remained in the diet (yes, you might have to give up ice cream and dairy for a while) or they continued taking calcium supplements. As in the case of all hormones, including D, we don't want to be deficient, but we don't want to overdo it either. *We have to know* our levels of intracellular calcium as well as our blood levels of D hormone to supplement correctly.

Calcium's link with osteoarthritis

Joint pain, bone aches, what's the difference? Well, there is a difference, but the underlying problems are closely linked. We're sure you got the answer right this time: excess calcium and mineral deficiencies. Take a moment to look back at the Calcium Cascade from Chapter 2. When your body tries to hold onto magnesium to protect the muscles and the heart and to compensate for the calcium excess, the adrenal glands are suppressed and sodium and potassium are lost in the urine. These essential mineral levels fall, further contributing to a relative calcium excess.

As these ratios keep going up and up and up, they create a downstream ripple effect that can become a flash flood. The adrenal glands are suppressed and the body's cells become increasingly resistant to thyroid hormone (type 2 hypothyroidism) and adrenal hormones. Think about the effects of calcium building up in places where it doesn't belong, whether it is in excess in the bones as spurs or calcific nodules, in the arteries as plaque, in the eyes as cataracts, in the cartilage as joint deterioration, in the connective tissues and arterial walls, or the kidneys and the gall bladder as stones. These problems are all clear warnings that you need an immediate HTMA test to accurately assess your dietary and supplement needs.

If you have excess calcium, it is building up in your body. Your connective tissues become weakened from inadequate protein digestion, and cell membrane electrical potential changes occur, which affect the all-important intracellular levels of calcium, sodium, magnesium and potassium (See

Chapter 4). This tissue weakness is further exacerbated by vitamin C deficiency (See Chapter 7). Deficiencies and imbalances of other essential minerals and amino acids also will impair the healing process. (More about this in Chapter 4.)

Osteocyte cells are responsible for the normal production of bone matrix, but when they lay down new bone over calcium deposits in the joint spaces, we get knobs, protrusions and deformed joints. This process is very complex and many other factors are at play. Calcium excess is the major underlying factor in joint deterioration, regardless of the pathway.

Osteoarthritis is the result of calcium-laden tissues in the joints. When you have too much calcium in the tissue, crystals or gravel begin to form, creating inflammation. Inflammation creates an abnormal healing response, and, as this calcium is deposited in your joints, you'll get creaking, grinding and bone spurs (new bone formation in an abnormal location), and increasing joint deformity results.

This problem may be increased by the use of the mineral strontium due to its natural function, that is, to interfere with excess calcium in the body. Strontium is often used incorrectly in Europe and less often in the U.S. to try to help treat osteoporosis. This is fundamentally and scientifically wrong. If calcium is high, strontium will almost always be high in the cells. Strontium becomes elevated with calcium to try to protect the body from the calcium excess.

It is more likely that strontium will cause abnormal bone formation as it incorporates itself into the bone remodeling process instead of calcium. It is one of those substituting minerals according to the principle I mentioned earlier, the Thompson-Döbereiner Theory of Mineral Substitution. This leads to abnormal and less resorptive bone crystals and impaired bone remodeling with resulting joint knobs and spurs in areas where there is the greatest bone turnover, the hands and feet. Strontium is unlikely to ever have any reliable positive scientific effect on the treatment osteoporosis. In my experience, strontium is never needed. Merely correcting calcium deficiency will correct strontium deficiency. It appears to be a following mineral, not a leader. Accordingly, when calcium is in excess, strontium is almost always in excess, too.

We know that osteoarthritis is not exclusively caused by "gravel" in the joints or by inflammation. It's also a process of the loss of collagen or soft

tissues like cartilage from amino acid deficiencies, vitamin C complex deficiency, impaired metabolism and impaired collagen production. The result
is chronic inflammation and tissue injury because your natural healing
response has gone awry. This can put you at risk for other inflammatory
health problems also related to calcium excess.

You probably won't be surprised to learn that the loss of collagen is also
related to excess calcium, partly because the amino acids that help build
these key soft tissues aren't being properly digested or absorbed. (See the
Calcium Cascade in Chapter 2 and the discussion of cell membrane electrical failure in Chapter 4.) Collagen itself is a fibrous protein that makes up
not only cartilage, but all the connective tissue in your body. Poor protein
absorption and poor digestion along with a deficiency of true vitamin C,
not ascorbic acid, directly affect collagen production and connective tissue
strength. Protein cannot be digested nor can the building-block amino acids
be absorbed into our cells without sodium and a proper mineral balance.

Your body cannot make collagen efficiently without copper in perfect
proportions with zinc. In order for copper to be present in the correct
amounts, your zinc levels must perfectly match it. Too much zinc interferes
with the copper needed to keep those soft tissues regenerating perfectly. We
also need a copper-carrying protein, a piece of the vitamin C complex molecule called tyrosinase, to help us use our bodies' copper supplies efficiently
so we can make collagen, hemoglobin, thyroid hormone, metabolize cholesterol and many more functions. (See Chapter 7.)

So if you can't properly digest those proteins because of mineral deficiency and you can't get that copper into your system or utilize it because of
vitamin C complex deficiency, collagen production and connective tissue
strength suffers. You can see how the cascade of ill effects continues. Much
of the degenerative disease of our joints, back and ligaments could be prevented with adequate real vitamin C (not "as ascorbic acid") intake and
replacing our true mineral needs.

Mineral balance is necessary for the proper absorption of vitamins,
amino acids and other nutrients. Vitamins as we know them in their "drug"
form cannot be used to form strong and healthy joint-stabilizing collagen.
Interestingly, our connective tissue should be stronger than bone. This is
not what we see due to the real vitamin C depletion by ascorbic acid, which
is commonly believed to be vitamin C. (See Chapter 7.)

It's the growing mineral imbalance and nutritional deficiencies, not the passing of the years, that make people more vulnerable to osteoarthritis and other degenerative and inflammatory diseases.

Just remember, we are talking about whole-food natural sources of these vitamins, not chemically or even "naturally" derived versions that only contain a part of the complex structure of the whole-food nutrients. We won't belabor this right now, but there will be lots more about The Vitamin Lie in Chapter 7.

It's easy to translate this excess calcium to other painful "gravelly" conditions like calcific plaque, cataracts, gallstones and kidney stones as well.

Those calcium crystals can build up in any soft tissue. They are often found in blood vessels, tissues and organs such as the heart, kidneys, brain, skin, joints, breast, eyes, liver, prostate and ovaries. Not only do these calcium deposits get bigger over time, they also trigger inflammation and other immune responses.

Other recent research shows the link between coronary heart disease, breast arterial calcification and bone mineral density. Calcium deposits in the arteries show the presence of atherosclerosis (commonly known as hardening of the arteries). Breast arterial calcification is often found in women with severe hardening of the arteries.

Abnormal soft tissue calcification happens when calcium binds with phosphate to form hard and bony structures, when calcium crystals accumulate in the wrong places, anywhere but in bones and teeth.

Isn't there calcium in sea salt and in these ionic minerals, too?

Yes, there is calcium in sea salt and in the balanced ionic trace mineral supplement I recommend. However, the calcium that is naturally occurring in these substances is in a specifically ordained balance with the other minerals. These trace minerals comprise about 15 percent of sea salt naturally. The supplement with the sodium essentially removed, as in the product that I recommend, represents 100 percent-balanced trace ionic minerals. What's important is the *balance* of calcium with other minerals in the rock salt and ionic salt form balanced trace minerals.

We'll repeat here: Calcium is a very important mineral in our bodies. I call it the "mineral king," but too much calcium causes serious health problems and almost all of us have too much intracellular and intercellular calcium. We all need calcium in our bodies, but we need it in the proper proportions to all the other minerals. The vast majority of us aren't getting those minerals in the proper proportions, so we're compromising not only our bones and joints, but also our entire well-being. Keep thinking minerals. Press the delete button on those outdated notions about calcium.

What to do if you've been diagnosed with osteoporosis

Your first step should be to get a hair tissue mineral analysis (HTMA) so you and your doctor will have a complete picture of your mineral status, showing the most essential mineral levels, toxic elements and the essential mineral ratios that affect your metabolism, digestion, thyroid, hormones, adrenals, muscles, hemoglobin and overall health.

You and your doctor can order HTMA from www.traceelements.com, through my website at www.calciumlie.com or through my office at 907-260-6914.

TEI is the only laboratory that I recommend at this time because of its high integrity, long record of excellence, huge database, personalized service, accurate reporting of essential mineral ratios that other laboratories don't even understand or report and most importantly, it's overall high level of accuracy and reproducibility. This laboratory has the USDA's CLIA certification, assuring its reliability in testing standards and results.

The results of the HTMA come with an assessment of the risk of a variety of health problems and temporary dietary and supplement change recommendations to minimize the likelihood of developing these problems or help in truly improving health. No other test that I have ever seen has more importance to our overall health. It goes without saying, follow those dietary recommendations. Although based on my experience with the HTMA testing, I frequently modify these recommendations to fit the patients' specific needs or clinical picture. But the only way—*the only way*—to improve your bone density and prevent osteoporosis reliably is to replace all the missing minerals that are responsible for bone strength and density in the correct proportions.

I'll say at the outset, it is very difficult to increase bone mineral density. It takes time and consistent mineral intake at levels of over 3 grams of balanced ionic trace minerals every day. Ionic sea salt-derived balanced trace minerals, however, will help stop the loss of those essential minerals if we adequately replace them.

It takes time for bone mineral density to increase. Anything over a 1.5 percent to 2 percent increase of bone density with correct mineral supplementation is highly significant. That is the minimum increase I see in most of the patients I treat with ionic sea salt-derived trace minerals. However in my most compliant and motivated patients, I often see increases that are as much as 8 percent per year.

The proper diet should not be ignored in this equation. Dramatically reducing or eliminating dairy products is probably the first positive step, and depending on your HTMA results, avoiding fatty meats, roasted nuts and certain heated oils, and increasing your intake of unrefined carbohydrates and certain specific vegetables may also be recommended. (See Chapter 9.)

Weight-bearing exercise is also an important element of increasing bone strength. This means walking, running, tennis, strength training or any activity that keeps you on your feet.

Gardening is one of Kathleen's favorite weight-bearing exercises, although most of us may not think of it that way. You actually get a better workout gardening than you do running—including calorie burn—because you're using all your large muscle groups, including the upper body.

I like walking, hiking, cross-country skiing, snowshoeing, mountain climbing and exercise that creates peace.

Walking is the absolute best way of all to decrease stress, improve health and stimulate growth in personal relationships. Kathleen and I both vote for walking as our favorite form of exercise. Kathleen wears a pedometer at all times and walks 10,000 steps a day or more. (More about that in chapter 9.)

POINTS TO REMEMBER

✔ Your body needs **at least 13 minerals** to build strong bones. Calcium is only one of them.

✔ My clinical experience shows that at least **90 percent of us are mineral deficient and have calcium excess**. This can actually weaken bones.

✔ Bone density tests are not very helpful because they are an average for people of your age, and as more and more people get osteopenia and osteoporosis, the lower the averages becomes. You should aim for the bone density of a healthy 20-year-old's bones.

✔ To expect bone and tissue mineral levels to decline with age is a mistaken conclusion. This decline is merely the result of nutritional mineral deficiency across our entire aging population.

✔ It's easier to prevent bone loss with adequate mineral supplementation, proper diet and exercise, than to try to rebuild lost bone mass.

✔ A hair tissue mineral analysis (HTMA) test, available through www.calciumlie.com or my office will give you the information you need to correct mineral imbalances and deficiencies, and begin to accurately address and prevent the health conditions these imbalances and deficiencies are causing.

CHAPTER 4

Digestive Dilemmas: Poor Protein Digestion, Sodium Deficiency and Cell Membrane Dysfunction

HAVE YOU NOTICED A TOUCH OF HEARTBURN now and then? Depending on your age, heartburn, gas, bloating and constipation may be unwelcome daily companions. Perhaps those calcium-rich Tums have a permanent place in your medicine cabinet. Maybe you think you get relief from Prilosec or Prevacid or you've even gone beyond over-the-counter digestive "aids" and you use other medications like Nexium, Tagamet or Zantac to control your symptoms. Or even worse, you use other medications like Maalox or Mylanta, which are full of toxic aluminum.

Probably you think of this problem as a minor nuisance. Maybe it's even a fairly major pain in the belly, but it's not serious, is it?

Yes, indeed, heartburn is very serious. It is often the first sign of a major system failure that can lead to a baffling cascade of deadly health problems. Neither you nor your doctors should dismiss heartburn and gastric upsets as "minor."

Fortunately, there is a great deal you can do to stop the downhill health slide that begins with heartburn.

Warning: Here comes some more biochemistry. It's crucial or we wouldn't put it here. We'll make it as simple and painless as possible.

Digestive distress can lead to serious trouble

Your doctor probably has told you that you have "acid indigestion" or "heartburn" or perhaps more formally GERD (gastroesophageal reflux disease), and that it is caused by excess acid production in your stomach. This is another of those nearly unshakeable erroneous belief systems that the medical community and the public seem to have embraced.

It stands to reason that excess acid is splashing up into your esophagus and causing a burning sensation, right?

That's only part of the story! What's really happening is that we cannot properly digest our food because we do not have *enough* stomach acid being released at the right time to do the job properly.

According to Dr. Jonathan Wright, author of *Why Stomach Acid is Good for You* (Evans, 2001), true acid over-production is extremely rare. But low acid production, causing just the symptoms of which 44 million of us, nearly one-third of all adults, complain at least once a month, is very common. Dr. Wright says stomach acid is essential to digestion and to the absorption of many vital nutrients, including protein and minerals.

MEDICAL FACT #1:
Stomach acid production declines with age.
MEDICAL FACT #2:
Heartburn and GERD increase with age. More than 50 percent of people over 50 complain of GERD.

So how could excess stomach acid production possibly be responsible for heartburn? It's not, or at least it's not what you think.

Doctors, even highly trained gastroenterologists, don't see the fallacy of putting patients on drugs called proton pump inhibitors that slow or even stop acid production. Worse yet, they don't think about the downstream effects of additional digestive problems. They don't realize that seemingly unrelated diseases like hypertension, depression, anxiety, migraines and insomnia are related to the failure of stomach acid production. These doctors have forgotten their basic medical biochemistry and physiology training.

In order to produce stomach acid (hydrochloric acid), the body needs sodium chloride. Right—salt. Sodium chloride is the body's only major natural source of chloride, the source of hydrochloric acid in the stomach's acid-producing cells, called parietal cells. That's why some divine wisdom has created sea salt at 85 percent sodium chloride and 15 percent other minerals—exactly what we need in exactly the right proportions.

But decades of medical badgering have caused most of us to rein in our salt intake to the point where the vast majority of us—more than 90 percent of my patients—are sodium deficient.

Don't be confused. Calcium excess also causes sodium and potassium loss in the urine and a continuous depletion of the intracellular stores of sodium and potassium. Remember the Calcium Cascade in Chapter 2? Potassium is also essential for the production of stomach acid. Most commonly, however, inadequate salt intake is a major factor.

I suspect that this holds true for almost everyone in the Western world who believes another nutritional lie that I call The Sodium Lie. Time and time again, I hear, "I don't use much salt." This is a big mistake! The result: We are losing our digestive abilities and more importantly, we're losing the ability to produce stomach acid correctly, the ability to digest protein, the ability to get amino acids into our cells and the ability to produce protein molecules, neurotransmitters and nitric oxide, leading to a whole host of nutrition-related diseases. All because we "cut back on salt." Just like all mammals, we need the (right kind of) salt!

Going back to the Calcium Cascade, we are reminded that excess calcium causes adrenal suppression so the kidneys can "grab" onto magnesium to balance out the excess calcium. Furthermore, when the adrenal glands are suppressed, there is a continuous loss of sodium and potassium in the urine, draining much-needed sodium and potassium from every cell in our bodies.

The loss of sodium and potassium reduces our ability to produce stomach acid, leading to an inability to digest protein and to use the amino acids that are essential to the majority of our body functions.

Now here's another problem: Many people eat Tums like candy when they're experiencing heartburn. What are Tums made of? Calcium. Oh, no! This means you're getting more calcium that will contribute to your problems by accelerating your intracellular sodium depletion exactly when you don't need it. In order for your body to absorb amino acids, you need sufficient stomach acid and sodium chloride. Low stomach acid allows those excess calcium molecules to roam around your body, depositing gravel-like residues into places where you don't want them—like in your arteries or joints. You certainly don't want that! This calcium excess is also like poison to the brain.

When the cells lining the lower part of the stomach or the upper part of the small intestine receive protein for digestion, they send signals to the acid-producing cells of the stomach through an increase in a hormone called gastrin. This hormone tells the stomach's parietal cells to start pro-

Calcium Cascade to Impaired Protein Digestion, Amino Acid Deficiency

DIETARY CALCIUM EXCESS

Adrenal suppression for magnesium retention

Urinary loss of sodium and potassium and inadequate intake of salt

Intracellular sodium and potassium depletion
(sodium/potassium membrane electrical potential failure)

Impaired, delayed, deficient stomach acid production

Poor protein digestion and absorption

Amino acid deficiencies and inability to get amino acids into our cells

Metabolic consequences, symptoms, disease

ducing or increase acid production. It's like the carburetor start-up system of an old car motor pumping the gas to try to get the engine started. If the acid doesn't come (like the car not starting), more pumping of the gas pedal is necessary. Eventually, if the engine doesn't start right away, continued pumping of the gas pedal occurs and the carburetor system gets flooded. Even if you're too young to remember these older cars, you get the picture.

Heartburn occurs in much the same way: As with the carburetor and an engine failing to start, too much pumping (gastrin stimulation to get the needed acid to digest protein), leads to flooding (too much acid being released all at once because of the overstimulation of acid-producing parietal cells). This has to occur because there was not enough acid production to begin the digestion of the protein meal when it first arrived in the stomach. We call this a paradoxical or indirect increased stomach acid production, because there is actually a deficiency first that leads to the excess later.

This again is due to the sodium deficiency in the acid-producing parietal cells lining the stomach, which require sodium chloride to do their work. The stomach thus becomes flooded; too much acid is finally released, too late and all at once, so you get heartburn.

This increased acid production can also be associated with high sodium levels inside the cells, resulting in a direct increase in acid or a continuous overproduction. Although this form of acid excess heartburn is less common, affecting less than 10 percent of those individuals with heartburn, it may be more severe. These patients are pouring out the acid due to excess intracellular sodium and stress factors. (See Chapter 9.) These are likely the patients who may be most prone to distal esophagitis, a risk factor for esophageal cancer.

Those with high cellular sodium levels confirmed by reliable HTMA results, unlike the vast majority of acid reflux sufferers, must restrict their sodium intake. They may also need prescription medications to help stop the acid stream until the problem is reversed. Stress management is a vitally important part of the treatment for people with high cellular sodium. (See Chapter 9.)

Once again, you and your doctor must know for certain the intracellular mineral concentrations in order to find relief and promote healing. All diet and medication recommendations must be based on knowing the body's intracellular mineral concentrations.

Conventional medical treatment for GERD symptoms usually leads us to "progress" to the need for prescription pharmaceuticals that are designed to halt the production of stomach acid. They work quite effectively, for all practical purposes, shutting down your acid production completely. How can you possibly digest protein or absorb the nutrients essential to your survival if you cannot digest your food? You can't!

Low stomach acid production causes incomplete digestion. Most importantly, proteins are not broken down into the amino acids we need to fuel trillions of body functions and make protein molecules in all the cells of the body. Minerals are not being absorbed properly or in the optimal ratios so our bodies start to malfunction. Bloating, gas and constipation often result from the poor protein digestion, especially after increased protein intake.

By the way, GERD is not exclusive to older adults. I've seen it in teenagers, especially in obese teens and even in 10-year-olds who invariably have intracellular calcium excess and severe sodium deficiency on HTMA results.

So what happens when you can't efficiently digest protein and get those crucial amino acids into the cells where they do their work?

The 20 standard amino acids include 8 essential amino acids and 4 semi-essential amino acids, which are needed to help your body to function. Without them, you're in trouble.

Here's a list of amino acids for those who like to delve more deeply into the subject.

AMINO ACIDS			
ESSENTIAL	**SEMI-ESSENTIAL**	**SOMETIMES ESSENTIAL**	**OTHERS**
Isoleucine	Arginine	Glutamine	Alanine
Leucine	Tyrosine	Glycine	Asparagine
Lysine	Cysteine	Proline	Aspartate
Methionine	Histidine	Serine	Glutamate
Phenylalanine			
Threonine			
Tryptophan			
Valine			

Let's talk first about amino acids that help us make neurotransmitters or brain chemicals:

Tryptophan is an essential amino acid that helps create the feel-good brain chemical serotonin. If poor protein digestion keeps your body from absorbing and utilizing tryptophan, the results can be depression, migraines, insomnia, anxiety, PMS, seasonal affective disorder (SAD) and even weight gain because of increased appetite and inability to sense when you have eaten enough. Phenylalanine, a substance found in artificial sweeteners, can interfere with the bioavailability of tryptophan and interfere with serotonin formation, with the same consequences as a deficiency in tryptophan. Tryptophan also makes niacin, vitamin B3, which helps your body rid itself of bad cholesterol.

5-Hydroxytryptophan (5-HTP) is the food-source amino acid form of tryptophan from which your body makes serotonin. It has been used quite effectively as a treatment for depression, anxiety, insomnia and migraine headaches when taken correctly.

Melatonin, another neurotransmitter hormone produced from tryptophan, helps regulate sleep cycles. Correction of this neurotransmitter deficiency also helps relieves sleep disorders and depression and is helpful as an antioxidant, neutralizing the deterioration of brain cells and reducing aging of the brain.

Interestingly the correct and most effective dose of melatonin is 200 mcg or 0.2 mg under the tongue or in a nasal spray. For international travel, up to 400 mcg doses are helpful. Just like any hormone, a transmucosal application, bypassing the liver, is the most effective form of delivery. Too much melatonin increases cortisol production, which then interferes with sleep. I recommend a 100 mcg per spray bottle; this dose would represent 2 sprays sublingual at bedtime. If you cannot obtain this low and most effective dose, splitting a 1 mg tablet into quarters and placing the small piece under the tongue until it dissolves is a close equivalent.

Think of all the drugs used to treat the symptoms of serotonin deficiencies that are associated with migraines, depression and anxiety. You've undoubtedly seen numerous television commercials about Prozac, Paxil, Celexa, Zoloft, Cymbalta and Lexapro to treat depression, Ambien, Lunesta and Sonata to treat insomnia and Amerge, Frova, Imitrex, Zomig and Maxalt for migraines, to name just a few of the multitude of pharmaceuticals used to treat conditions resulting from serotonin deficiency caused in most cases by low tryptophan absorption and utilization.

With about 30 million people in the U.S.—about 8 percent of the population—showing signs of clinical depression at any given time, there is a multibillion dollar market for these drugs. In fact, almost all of these sufferers can be treated successfully with food and correct supplements without these potentially harmful and expensive drugs. Recognizing and correcting thyroid issues can also be very helpful. (See Chapter 5.)

Do you really think your body has a Zoloft or Lunesta or Imitrex deficiency? How absurd is that thinking? Your body needs more minerals and more minerals in balance and, in most cases, more sea salt. That will result in better protein digestion and more amino acids available to your cells to make the brain chemicals you need to stay mentally healthy. Also, remember 95 percent of our neurotransmitters are found in the gastrointestinal tract. This may be why we get "gut feelings." Nearly all the neurotransmitters in the body (chemical communicators for the nervous system) are derived from amino acids. Many GI problems may be in part related to these neurotransmitter deficiencies. We need to treat the underlying problem, not just the symptoms!

Jenny's Story

Jenny was only 11 when I first met her. As she and her mother sat in my office, Jenny was thin and pale. She certainly looked glum for an 11-year-old. Her mom was clearly at the end of her rope.

Jenny had blinding migraine headaches virtually every day for over five years. The situation was so bad that she rarely was able to stay in school past noon. That's not much of a life for a sixth grader who should have been playing soccer, marching in the school band or ice skating in winter. Jenny had become a virtual invalid in this day of "highly advanced" modern medicine.

Her concerned parents had sought the best possible medical attention for Jenny. She had been to every neurologist in the state of Alaska and even to specialized medical clinics in Washington and Minnesota. Despite a battery of every test known to medicine and a medicine chest full of prescription drugs, nothing was helping Jenny.

I recognized that Jenny was suffering from sodium deficiency, poor digestion and membrane electrical failure from mineral imbalances resulting in tryptophan amino acid deficiency. As a result, her body was unable to digest, absorb and utilize the proteins and amino acids that would help her manufacture serotonin. It wasn't a surprise that she had migraines and perhaps a little depression, too.

I started Jenny on minerals and a regimen of supplements to help her replace her neurotransmitters and ordered a hair tissue mineral analysis (HTMA) that confirmed what I suspected: She had excess calcium and low sodium in her tissues.

But even before the HTMA results came back, Jenny had made a dramatic turnaround. In just four days, her migraines had disappeared! She and her mom both hugged me for joy. There wasn't a dry eye in my office. All that poor little girl needed was a few minerals and the right high-quality nutritional supplements.

She was weaned off her medications (you can't stop most of these medications cold turkey without causing some potentially terrible results).

Eight years later, Jenny is still headache free, as long as she continues to take her minerals and supplements. She is now a happy and well-adjusted teenager who told me on her last visit she had just entered her sophmore year in college.

I learned recently that Jenny's pediatrician had pooh-poohed my treatment and said that Jenny probably "just grew out of her migraines." In four days? This is intellectual dishonesty. This physician should have asked if he could use or apply these treatments with his other patients. He obviously had no interest in getting Jenny better and even less interest in learning how to better care for his patients. It's sad, but too commonly true in today's medicine.

Jenny and her family know better and they're unlikely to trust conventional doctors for a long time to come. Why wouldn't a caring physician want to learn what worked, why it worked and if it could help their other patients? It is amazing to me that these doctors are not interested or just don't care enough to really help their patients get better. Patients do not care how much the doctor knows, they care how much the doctor cares. It follows intuitively: caring doctors know more.

Tyrosine is a semi-essential amino acid necessary for the body to create the anti-stress hormones dopamine and norepinephrine. Tyrosine is also an essential part of the manufacture of the proteins that make insulin receptors, which keep blood sugars steady, and of thyroid hormones that regulate metabolic rate and energy levels. It's also a part of the process that creates coenzyme Q10, a vital part of the body's energy production machinery that also plays a role in creating (good) cholesterol and governing muscle function. It's easy to see the effects of an inability to absorb and utilize tyrosine on adrenal function and other biological functions.

Methionine is another essential amino acid vital to the body's metabolism for detoxification, energy production and enzymatic activities, including those that govern digestion, among many other things. Methionine is the spark plug that tells the cells to duplicate themselves perfectly, thereby preventing the cell deterioration that results in aging. Graying hair and deteriorating eyesight mean your cells are not duplicating themselves as perfectly as they did when you were young. Methionine is a critical element in keeping those cells identical, generation after generation. In its natural state, methionine is a methyl donor, very important to our cellular biochemistry, energy production, DNA structure, gene expression, homocysteine metabolism, and as methylsulfonylmethane (MSM), it contains a sulfur atom that helps our bodies detoxify and excrete heavy metals.

Arginine is another amino acid with far-reaching metabolic effects. It is necessary for your body to produce nitric oxide, a vasodilator or blood vessel expander that signals your circulatory system that it is time to relax and expand. Without nitric oxide, blood vessels become constricted, blood flow is diminished and high blood pressure or hypertension results. Patients with chest pain are often given nitroglycerin to help relax blood vessels. Arginine has similar results over a longer period of time. Arginine is also important in wound healing, cellular division, peripheral circulation, penile erections, immune function, the release of hormones (including growth hormone), and it helps with removal of toxic ammonia from the body. It is also important in the formation of myelin protein, nerve regeneration, RNA processing and transcription, DNA repair, immune function and prevention of autoimmune diseases.

Arginine is also necessary for the body to make creatine, a naturally—occurring energy source for muscle and nerve cells. Creatine is used commonly to enhance muscle performance (safe up to 3 grams per day) and is used medically as supportive therapy in neuromuscular diseases.

Large doses of arginine are commonly being recommended today in diabetic patients to help with blood vessel dilatation and to improve peripheral circulation. This is mediated by the increase in nitric oxide produced from arginine. But remember, arginine cannot enter into our cells, and therefore nitric oxide production cannot occur without sodium.

Carnitine, an amino acid found primarily in meat products, is a key component of your body's energy production. Carnitine is like a train that transports fats to the mitochondria, the body's energy furnaces, where the fats are burned as fuel. Carnitine also helps sweep toxins out of the body and helps regulate cholesterol.

Glycine is important for the production of hemoglobin, the oxygen carrying protein molecule in red blood cells. It also combines with cysteine and glutamic acid in the body to form glutathione, an important antioxidant in the body. This amino acid is also a methyl donor and very important to our metabolism, cellular biochemistry and physiology.

Lysine is an amino acid that is an important element of energy production, by a process called methylation that allows the donation of methyl groups for every organic biochemical reaction in our bodies to take place. It's also important for the formation of collagen for healthy joints and skin.

Serine is important to the activation of many enzymes, another type of bodily "spark plug" that sets off chemical reactions. These enzymes do everything, from digesting food to transporting molecules across cell membranes, so they can be used for energy. It is also important in the formation of numerous substances that sustain brain function. The improper absorption of serine has been implicated in the onset of type 2 diabetes.

Threonine is an amino acid that is important in protein formation and in the formation of the processes that keep your energy furnaces burning.

Of the other essential amino acids, many have less obviously critical roles and are principally involved in the production of protein molecules to sustain vital biological functions throughout the body.

Other important amino acid molecules include the "nonstandard" amino acids that are not found in protein molecules in the body, but may act alone to turn on, turn off, carry on, carry out and facilitate biochemical reactions in the body, such as GABA (gamma-aminobutyric acid), glycine and glutamate. These are all very important brain chemicals.

We've given you this list of some of the more important amino acids so you can see that a deficiency of any amino acid could have far-reaching implications to our health and longevity.

Impaired protein and amino acid digestion and sodium deficiency are major factors leading to many diseases.

Sodium/Potassium Membrane Electrical Dysfunction (S/PMEP)

We wish we could tell you that digestive malfunction was the end of this complex biochemical chain that causes health problems but, in truth, it's just the beginning.

Warning: Here's some more biochemistry. Skip this if you like, but it *is* important.

Excess calcium causes adrenal suppression with a resulting continuous loss of large amounts of sodium and potassium in the urine, even though our bodies are desperately seeking additional sources of these two essential minerals to ensure a steady heartbeat, so that muscle and nerve fibers will fire when they are needed and blood pressure stays stable.

Excess calcium and the resulting deficiencies in intracellular sodium and potassium cause a failure of the sodium/potassium membrane electrical

A Primer on Biological Methylation
(Made as Simple as Possible)

Methylation is the process of donating or removing a CH3 bond (carbon and three hydrogen atoms) from one substance to another to facilitate the biochemistry of our bodies. From a metabolic standpoint, these substances may be the next most important substances we put into our bodies after water and trace minerals. I often say they are the other half of our biologic metabolic equation. Minerals are electron donors and methyl carriers are methyl donors. They are found in fresh food. These methyl groups are transferred by enzymes called methlytransferases.

Biochemical processes requiring transmethlylation include histamine metabolism, methionine cycle, adrenal function, brain neurotransmitter balance, myelin stability, estrogen metabolism, cell membrane structure, and liver detoxification to name a few.

Some amino acids are methyl donors naturally such as methyl-sulfa-methionine (MSM), dimethyl and trimethly-glycine (betaine HCL or TMG), tetra-methyl-lysine (TML), di-methyl-arginine, methyl-selenocysteine, S-adenosyl-methionine (SAMe), methyl-malonic acid, N-acetyl-5-meth-oxytryptamine (melatonin), and methyl-hydroxy-serine. Certain B vitamins are also very important in methylation including pyridoxine (B6, involved in the formation of neurotransmitters, serotonin and norepinephrine, myelin for nerve insulation and the conversion of tryptophan to niacinamide, fat metabolism, prostaglandin formation and magnesium utilization), 5-methyl-tetrahydrofolate (B9, one of the most important B vitamins of all, important in homocysteine metabolism) and methyl cyanocobalamin (B12).

Illnesses related to methyl deficiency include histamine imbalance illnesses such as asthma and allergic rhinitis, gastric acid formation problems, stress and inflammatory conditions, insulin resistance, depression, melatonin synthesis and deficiency problems, serotonin synthesis and deficiency problems such as depression and insomnia, myelin formation for nerve sheaths, cancer, estrogen metabolism, phosphotidylcholine formation for cell membranes, liver metabolism and reactions including sulfation, glucuronidation, acetylation, and amino acid metabolism and many more detoxification reactions.

Hypermethylation (too much methyl) has been associated with Parkinson's disease. It is difficult to know if this excess is a cause or an effect of the disease or its biochemical etiology.

I recommend supplementation with MSM as an excellent and inexpensive methyl donor to help insure adequate methylation. It is an essential amino acid nutrient with profound effects on well-being, increasing energy, detoxing heavy metals and increasing enzyme activity. I recommend at least 3 grams per day.

potential (S/PMEP) of the cell membranes of every cell in the human body, with far-reaching consequences. Interestingly, it is this electrical potential of every cell membrane in the body that is responsible for the pictures we get from magnetic resonance imaging, or MRI, studies.

The S/PMEP moves sodium out of cells and potassium into the cells. It is a negative electrical charge on the inside of the cell that ushers these minerals in and out of the cells. It is this mechanism (still today being incorrectly taught to biochemistry students as the "sodium pump") that keeps sodium out of the cells and potassium in, helping sodium atoms transport glucose, amino acids and other nutrients into the cells.

It's not hard to imagine, then, what happens when there is not enough sodium and potassium to maintain this cellular electrical membrane potential, thereby decreasing the body's ability to get amino acids and glucose into all our cells (except fat cells, which still absorb glucose directly without sodium). Basically, this results in cellular dysfunction and failure that has long-reaching consequences. If we can't get these amino acids into our cells, our bodies cannot grow and repair and carry on normal metabolism. Without glucose in organ and tissue cells, your body has no fuel for energy. That spells a serious energy problem for you and your body. (More about this in Chapter 5.)

In my practice, I've discovered that the average patient has only 5 to 20 percent of the normal intracellular sodium content and 7 to 15 percent of the needed intracellular potassium, even if blood tests are normal. That's why I tell my patients, with confidence based on 13 years of experience and nearly 2000 HTMA results, that they are making a big mistake at least 90 percent of the time when they boast that they "hardly eat any salt."

Amino acid deficiency means your body cannot grow and repair itself. Without these essential nutrients, your body will begin to cannibalize itself, sucking proteins from the muscles, brain, nerves and other organ tissues. The immune system is also compromised, so an early sign of amino acid deficiency may be increased vulnerability to infections. This vulnerability may be largely due to reduced adrenal function caused by the high calcium and severely depleted intracellular sodium levels. This is what we see in at least 90 percent of our tests. Lowered protein levels may also lead to edema, or fluid retention outside the cells, resulting in swollen ankles, hands or face.

Over the long term, those amino acid deficiencies can result in high blood pressure, heart disease, stroke, loss of immune system function, increased cancer risk, depression, anxiety, insomnia, migraine headaches and many more chronic medical problems. Undoubtedly, there are many more consequences of amino acid deficiencies that have not yet been documented because conventional medicine is so focused on the idea that disease means we need drugs or surgery. In developed countries, another myth is that most of us consume more protein than we need. Just because we're chowing down on steaks and burgers and getting loads of dietary protein doesn't mean we're able to assimilate the nutrients in the protein.

Medical science doesn't want to believe we could be amino acid deficient when we eat so much protein. Again, we're looking at basic college biochemistry. Science doesn't lie, but humans seem to be very susceptible to unscientific ideas about the biochemical functions of the human body.

Doctors (and the rest of us, too) need to take another look at the biochemistry textbooks and apply those basic scientific concepts to the practice of medicine. We need to be sure that our doctors are not practicing medicine as a religion based on a belief in some erroneous concepts, rather than on hard scientific facts, e.g., The Calcium Lie. Remember, Hippocrates said, "To know is good science, to believe one knows is ignorance." We have to *know* our mineral content, levels, imbalances and deficiencies to correct them and prevent the disease catastrophes we see today.

It also shouldn't be shocking to learn that S/PMEP failure has been associated with calcium leaking into cells that overload with calcium, which can lead to heart failure, cardiac arrhythmia, hypothyroidism (type 2, see Chapter 5), hypertension, dementia from brain shrinkage and synapse dysfunction, kidney stones and failure, and many more excess calcium related problems. The Calcium Lie quickly becomes an even more serious problem when the immune system is compromised. We must quit thinking calcium alone and start thinking minerals are what we need.

Hypertension (high blood pressure) is often treated with drugs called calcium channel blockers, angiotensin II receptor blockers (ARBs) and angiotensin-converting enzyme (ACE) inhibitors, beta blockers, alpha blockers, and diuretics. All of these are intended to relax constricted blood vessels and treat the hypertension. Think about this: They are called calcium channel blockers because . . . ? The answer is simple: They're blocking the effects of the excess calcium going into the cells.

It's time for us to wake up and realize that excess calcium is a major factor in hypertension and heart disease. Worse yet, these calcium channel blockers have numerous side effects, including muscle aches, dizziness, headache, fluid buildup in the legs and feet, constipation, slow heart rate, and flushing. In my experience, these side effects are made worse by sodium depletion.

For the past several years, the U.S. and Europe have endured record-breaking high summer temperatures. Elderly people are particularly vulnerable to heat exhaustion and death, especially those with heart disease whose doctors routinely put them on sodium-restricted diets. In my opinion, these people die needlessly because their low-sodium diets have made them sodium and potassium depleted and less likely to respond to resuscitation efforts.

In November of 2007, doctors at the National Institutes of Health convened to discuss further reduction in the recommended daily salt intake. We certainly aren't learning from history. Recommending general sodium restriction when 90 percent of us need *more* sodium is just bad medicine bordering on malpractice. We need to know for sure who needs sodium and who should avoid it. It is not a "one size fits all."

Now think back to the Calcium Cascade for a moment. Better yet, look through the diagram in Chapter 2.

The adrenal suppression that results from the Calcium Cascade means that sodium and potassium, the exact minerals so desperately needed in our cells for the sodium/potassium membrane electrical potential to function, are being excreted in large amounts through the urine. When the body's stores of sodium and potassium are depleted, the body begins to shut down. Cellular energy production declines and calcium leaks into our cells too rapidly. The result: lack of energy, cardiac arrhythmia, plaque, stones, bone spurs, vascular disease, hypertension, dementia and thyroid hormone resistance or type 2 hypothyroidism, just to name a few.

Sorry, the bad news isn't over yet. Amino acids help build protein receptors on the cell walls. And guess what? Insulin receptors are made of protein molecules and minerals. If the amino acid deficiency caused by incomplete digestion of proteins compromises cellular function, the cells have fewer insulin receptors, so the cells can't balance blood glucose. We'll talk about insulin resistance more in Chapter 5, but for now you need to know that insulin resistance leads to type 2 diabetes and a whole host of increased risks for heart disease, kidney failure, nerve damage, improper wound healing, blindness, dementia, cancer and more. All of these effects of poor protein digestion, mineral deficiency and imbalance, and sodium/potassium membrane electrical potential failure add up to big trouble.

Prevention and treatment

It's a really ugly Gordian knot, but it's one that can be untied with some common sense. All of the illnesses associated with protein digestion failure and S/PMEP are preventable and treatable. All it takes is basic knowledge of biochemistry and human physiology, reliable HTMA results and correct supplementation, along with some basic whole-food and a better diet.

We must begin to re-examine how we treat many of these illnesses based on actual knowledge of mineral deficiency and imbalance effects on our body's biochemistry and metabolism. I am clearly suggesting that over 90 percent of all hypertension in the world is being treated incorrectly without this knowledge. We have to know our tissue mineral levels and critical ratios to decide with our doctors a plan of action. Every nutritional and medication recommendation needs to be based on knowing this information.

Depression, anxiety and insomnia

It's not a deficiency of Paxil or Prozac or Celexa that is causing depression. Depression is caused by an inability to produce the neurotransmitters you need to keep from being depressed. If you just trace back to the beginnings of acid indigestion, or the failure to digest and absorb proteins and transport amino acids into the cells, and the S/PMEP failure, you have the answers to prevention, treatment and elimination of symptoms of many serious diseases including depression and anxiety, obesity, type 2 diabetes, migraines, hypertension, dementia and type 2 hypothyroidism.

If these nutritional problems are treated correctly, in almost every case the disease or illness will disappear or lessen in severity over time, often reducing the need for medication. (More about this in Chapter 8.)

Taking action

1. The first thing: Get a hair tissue mineral analysis (HTMA) available

through www.calciumlie.com. This test will let you know your exact mineral status. Your intracellular sodium, calcium, magnesium and potassium levels and their ratios are especially important in determining your overall health; the effectiveness of your protein digestion, water- and acid-base balance, energy production, thyroid function, adrenal function; and a whole host of other medical problems. You will also get valuable information about toxic minerals and heavy metal levels and various trace mineral levels from the HTMA test.

2. Even while you're waiting for your HTMA results, begin to use more unrefined natural sea salt to help bring up your sodium levels. You can fairly safely assume your sodium levels are too low since there is a 90-percent chance. See the resource section for specific product recommen-dations or refer to our website, www.calciumlie.com, for the products I recommend. It takes both diet changes and supplements to correct a life-time of accumulated mineral deficiency and imbalance.

3. Begin to wean yourself off proton pump inhibitors and medication designed to lower your acid production. You may need the help of your doctor to do this—and you may get some serious resistance. Stick to your guns. Show your doctor this book and encourage him or her to recall college biochemistry and physiology. Your HTMA will tell you to be sure. There may be some exceptions in this group, in people with chronic distal esophagitis, or Barrett's esophagitis, considered in some cases to be precancerous and worsened by excess stomach acid.

4. If needed, I treat heartburn with DGL licorice, which absorbs the acid excess harmlessly without interfering with protein digestion. Correcting the intracellular sodium levels has a huge impact on reducing or elimi-nating this problem over time.

5. Start taking supplements and use more sodium if indicated; this will help retrain your stomach to produce acid more correctly. I also recommend Rhizonate, a form of licorice extract. Chew one every five minutes until you get relief. Over time, this is effective for almost everybody. It absorbs the excess acid harmlessly and still allows for some protein digestion.

6. If you're depressed, but you don't experience heartburn, you probably still have some degree of sodium deficiency. Try this: Take extra sea salt

and amino acids to correct the protein digestion deficiency and add 5-HTP (5-hydroxytryptophan), 150 to 600 mg at bedtime, to help re-establish and correct serotonin neurotransmitter production and bring up your serotonin levels. Once serotonin levels are corrected, maintenance doses of 100 to 150 mg will keep the doctor away.

7. If you also have anxiety and/or insomnia, additional and sometimes different amino acid supplements and nutritional corrections may be needed. In more complicated patients, with overlapping diagnoses, I also recommend specific neurotransmitter testing and replacement of the specific neurotransmitter-related amino acid deficiencies.

8. If you have high blood pressure, you'll need to treat as many of the underlying problems as possible. Get more arginine into your body to help with nitric oxide production. A sustained-release form is best due to the short half-life of arginine in the blood. I recommend one called Perfusia, available through the calciumlie.com website. It's also helpful to stop eating foods that contain gluten (gluten makes the red blood cells sticky). This includes nearly all wheat products, and I recommend we minimize or eliminate most dairy products.

9. Many people with incomplete protein digestion and S/PMEP failure also have essential fatty acid deficiencies, so a high-quality fish oil product is an important part of the healing process. Eicosamax is the ultrapure, heavy metal-free omega-3 product I recommend. Shark liver oil is exceptionally pure and is also very effective when used correctly, but is only available in limited amounts. (See Chapter 8 for more information on finding the best supplements.)

Marybeth's story

Marybeth wasn't unknown to me when I started treating her. She had been a friend and a colleague for quite some time, so I'd observed her over the course of several years. We had shared meals and I'd seen her distress after our families shared a zeal for Mexican food. At 52, she began to pay a heavy price for all that spicy food.

I'd watched her pop Tums over the years and then finally find a doctor who put her on a proton pump inhibitor. There was temporary relief from her intense heartburn, but the heartburn returned and she added Tums back to the prescription meds. She was a mess and the first to admit it!

I absolutely hated watching her suffer, but ethics prohibited me from offering help until I was asked.

"Can more medicine help?" she finally asked me.

"No," I answered immediately. "But less medicine may help you a lot."

She was willing to try.

I put her on an acid absorber (Rhizonate) instead of an acid inhibitor. I gave her a mineral supplement to restore her mineral balance based on HTMA results, and encouraged her to use unrefined sea salt liberally in her diet based on these results showing severe intracellular sodium deficiency. When Marybeth saw her tissue mineral analysis results and the documentation of her sodium depletion, she became a believer.

Relief didn't come overnight, but in the space of about three months, Marybeth was able to get off all her prescription meds. Over time, we were able to reverse her sodium deficiency and retrain her stomach to produce acid correctly. Six years later, Marybeth is still free of prescription meds and heartburn, unless she really goes overboard with the Mexican food. These days, when our families get together for a meal, we usually opt for something a little kinder to her digestive tract.

I have no doubt that in time, she will be completely free of the digestive symptoms that signaled that my friend was at high risk for many more serious health problems.

POINTS TO REMEMBER

✔ Heartburn, gas, bloating, constipation and general indigestion are often the first signs of problems related to mineral deficiencies and imbalances, poor protein digestion, sodium deficiency and calcium excess in over 90 percent of patients.

✔ Heartburn, also known as GERD (gastroesophageal reflux disease), is most often caused by low or inadequate stomach acid production, not the continuous presence of too much stomach acid.

✔ When there is insufficient stomach acid, proteins are not properly digested. The result is that amino acids, essential for many body metabolic processes, are not absorbed and, therefore, not available for metabolism, growth and repair and other body needs. Calcium excess and sodium deficiency problems lead to most amino acid deficiency-related medical problems.

✔ The sodium/potassium membrane electrical potential failure due to low intracellular sodium and potassium levels significantly impairs the absorption of life-giving amino acids and glucose into all our cells (except fat cells, which continue to absorb glucose independent of S/PMEP) and these cells continue to grow stimulated by an abundance of insulin, insulin resistance and increased glucose levels.

✔ Over the long term, amino acid deficiencies can result in medical problems including depression, anxiety, migraine headaches, hypothyroidism, metabolic syndrome, high blood pressure, heart disease, vascular disease, stroke, neuropathy, dementia, loss of immune system function and autoimmune diseases, increased cancer risk and more.

✔ S/PMEP failure has been clearly associated with too much calcium in the cells. Over time, this leads to many medical problems.

✔ We have to know for sure our intracellular mineral levels to prevent, accurately diagnose and correctly treat these illnesses. Medication and dietary recommendations are potentially flawed without a reliable HTMA results.

CHAPTER 5

Metabolic Failure

How Excess Calcium Causes Weight Gain, Thyroid and Adrenal Malfunctions, and Five Types of Hypothyroidism

PART 1: WEIGHT ISSUES

Are you overweight? Is someone you love overweight?

No doubt, your doctor has told you to eat less and exercise more while discreetly adjusting a lab coat to cover a personal paunch. Take a good look. Is your doctor an example of good health? If not, maybe you need a change.

It seems too simple. So you struggle. You faithfully get up at 5 a.m. every day for a morning jog or Zumba. You try Atkins, South Beach, Jenny Craig and Weight Watchers. You gulp down chromium picolinate, 5-HTP, garcinia cambogia, hoodia, Alli, green coffee, dark chocolate, raspberry ketones, and every other known fad weight-loss supplement. You've probably had some success, but for almost all of us, the success is temporary. The weight begins to creep back on until you've regained all you lost and then some.

Why is that? Are we all weak-willed, unable to resist the temptation of the dinner plate? Is our willpower so lacking that we can't even do the basic exercise of pushing away from the dinner table?

No! This answer may surprise you, but we are turning into a fat nation (Generation XL) because we are quite literally starving. That's right: In a time of unparalleled food wealth, we cannot get the nutrients from our food that our bodies need to function normally. Quite literally, our mineral deficiencies and imbalances, especially calcium excess, is leading us to metabolic failures of unprecedented proportions.

We know that sounds like an oxymoron, but you may be fat and also be starving. If you add up what you've learned in the first four chapters of this book, it will all start to make sense.

What are we starving for? You guessed it: Minerals. What are we stuffed with? We're sure you guessed it again: Calcium.

It's a vicious circle: We are starving for the minerals we need, and so we are driven, through cravings to eat more and more food in an effort to get those minerals into our cells where they are essential for literally trillions of metabolic functions, but our foods are low in minerals because of our mineral-poor soil and because few are vine ripened (Chapter 1). So we eat more and more. Our metabolisms are slowed because of calcium excess, adrenal suppression and thyroid hormone resistance (type 2 hypothyroidism; more about that shortly). Digestion is impaired; stomach acid is deficient or improperly released. Protein is not fully digested and essential amino acids are not absorbed. Amino acids can't make it into our cells due to sodium/potassium membrane electrical potential (S/PMEP) failure. More cravings are stimulated by amino acid and glucose deficiencies in all our cells (except fat cells) and the resulting neurotransmitter deficiencies (especially serotonin, which helps control appetite).

It's a terrible, uncontrollable, downward spiral. Since we all know the well-documented health risks of being overweight and the epidemic proportions of obesity in our population (nearly 60 percent in some states), it all seems so sad to think that we are killing ourselves in a desperate struggle to get the nutrients we need to survive and all the while we are admonished to watch our sodium, get our calcium and to diet and exercise.

So how does this all work?

Knowing that almost every single American is mineral deficient, it isn't a great leap of logic to think about deficiencies and imbalances in certain minerals causing cravings. Those cravings may be for sugary foods or they may be for salty foods or both.

Sugary food cravings probably mean you are becoming insulin resistant and entering into a state of unhealth called metabolic syndrome in which you have elevated insulin levels, high blood pressure, elevated total cholesterol and triglycerides, and obesity. This has sometimes been called "prediabetes" because, while your fasting blood sugars may still be within the normal range, you are almost inevitably headed toward full-blown and preventable type 2 diabetes and all of its side effects, including heart disease, stroke, kidney failure, poor circulation leading to amputations, macular degeneration, retinal hemorrhages leading to blindness and the list goes on and on.

Low blood sugar or hypoglycemia is actually caused by insulin resistance. When your glucose metabolism becomes impaired and you eat something sugary, say a donut (oh, horrors!) your body releases a load of insulin, overcompensating for the sugar and causing your blood sugar to drop. It's not surprising that your body then craves more sugar to try to bring your sugars back up, give you energy and a vicious cycle is born. This is a warning sign that type 2 diabetes is on its way into your life. Just losing weight doesn't treat the underlying problem, no matter which diet you choose. This physiology is subjecting huge numbers of people to what I call "the weight roller coaster."

Cravings for salty foods may also be related to insulin resistance, but these cravings along with cravings for fatty foods are even more directly linked to mineral deficiencies since so many minerals have salty flavors, including, of course, sodium.

Hmmm, salty, fatty food and sugar . . . a Quarter Pounder, fries and a Coke . . . No wonder McDonald's raked in $27.56 billion worldwide in 2012 from over 34,000 restaurants worldwide serving around 68 million customers daily in 119 countries. Add in all the other fast, fried and super-processed foods that are a regular part of our American diets and a pattern becomes clear.

Food cravings are basically a form of pica, which refers to an eating disorder that involves eating nonfood items, most commonly dirt, clay, cornstarch, laundry starch and baking soda. It is the body's attempt to get more minerals into the body and is most common in children and pregnancy. You'll probably be interested to know that as many at 68 percent of pregnant women develop some form of pica, but it is also fairly common among the rest of the population. This is interesting, since we know that each pregnancy drains 10 percent or more of a woman's total body mineral supply, so "pica" is the body's desperate attempt to replace those essential and missing minerals.

Adequate mineral supplementation with ionic sea salt-derived balanced trace minerals may, in fact, be the most important nutritional choice we can make to maintain normal weight as well as before, during and after pregnancy especially if breast-feeding. (See Chapter 6.)

Iron supplementation is the most common treatment for pica, so the mainstream medical community seems to have gotten the idea that this eating disorder is the result of the human's insatiable quest for iron for survival. But iron is not the only deficient mineral and iron deficiency is typically only a symptom of a greater imbalance in the body's mineral supplies, quite literally the tip of the iceberg. Very often, vitamin C deficiency is also a problem. The body cannot absorb iron or use it without the whole vitamin C molecule, not as ascorbic acid. (See Chapter 7.) This imbalance is often exaggerated by calcium supplementation, especially in women whose intracellular calcium levels are already too high.

We're here to tell you that if you exercise like a hamster on the wheel and eat nothing but lettuce for the rest of your life to lose weight, it will cause no permanent changes unless you treat your underlying metabolic issues and imbalances by balancing and raising your mineral levels and supplementing correctly. **All meaningful weight loss must involve treating and correcting the underlying metabolism.** This is even more critical for patients who have undergone weight reduction bypass procedures that may further accentuate mineral, amino acid and other nutritional deficiencies and imbalances.

Let's back up a little bit and define the metabolic failure that is the link between calcium excess, mineral deficiency and obesity.

Take a look at the Calcium Cascade in Chapter 2. You'll see the way that calcium excess leads to the failure of the body to respond to insulin to control blood glucose, the failure to produce energy efficiently through glycogen and most importantly, to the failure of thyroid hormones to be able to stimulate our metabolism.

Low thyroid hormone levels are not the only cause of obesity, but over 95 percent of all obese patients in my practice have hypothyroidism, due to calcium excess with thyroid hormone resistance (type 2 hypothyroidism), and the resulting metabolic failures.

This is what I call a **Nutritional Disease Cascade**. It goes like this:

NUTRITIONAL DISEASE CASCADE

1. Deficiency develops

Body nutrients (especially minerals) and essential amino acids are depleted,
and calcium is in excess in all the cells in the body, *SO*

2. Compensation occurs

Your body begins to have some subtle metabolic and biochemical changes,
but these are not yet detectable in laboratory blood tests. *THEN,*

You develop increasing thyroid hormone resistance, calcium-to-potassium intracellular imbalance, slowed metabolism and adrenal suppression, as your body attempts to hold on to magnesium to balance the high intracellular calcium to keep muscles and nerves working correctly. Decreased absorption of nutrients in foods occurs from poor digestion and lack of absorption of the nutrients, metabolism is slowed and sodium and potassium are continuously lost from your cellular reserves into your urine.

You lose the ability to produce stomach acid, leading to poor protein digestion and sodium/potassium membrane electrical potential failure, with a resulting inability to get essential amino acids and glucose into your cells, except fat cells, which are stimulated by the increasing insulin levels to absorb the extra glucose, and these fat cells remain independent of the sodium/potassium membrane potential, absorbing glucose by another process. Those fat cells continue to absorb more and more glucose and they grow larger and more numerous all the time.

As insulin sensitivity decreases or resistance develops, more insulin is needed
and with higher insulin levels, more fat is produced, *AND*

3. Un-compensation occurs

You begin to have slightly elevated triglyceride levels (over 100), slightly elevated blood sugars (91–124), and lowered G/I ratios (7–13 range) that show insulin resistance, but still changes are minor enough to escape much notice. It is not a crisis yet, so most people carry on. However, your body has begun to make fat more easily. You gain weight quickly and have increased difficulty losing weight due to the underlying mineral deficiencies and imbalances, thyroid hormone resistance and adrenal hormone resistance with further slowing of your metabolism and continued increases in insulin resistance.

You don't know how to treat it, so you eat less, diet and exercise, and your metabolism slows even more. You may, for a short time, maintain the weight loss, then you get back on the roller coaster and gain it all back because your body is still craving the nutrients it needs. This is a common problem with all current weight-loss programs and diets. *EVENTUALLY*

4. Clinical disease develops in two stages

Clinical disease develops, most likely type 2 diabetes, hypertension or a neurotransmitter (brain chemistry) disease like depression and anxiety or migraines. *In the early stages, it is:*

4a. Reversible clinical disease: It can be reversed by rebalancing and raising the mineral levels, correct supplementation based on HTMA results, by lowering the calcium excess if necessary, and possibly with the addition of extra thyroid hormone until the thyroid resistance problem corrects. You can tell by measuring basal body temperature until it is over 97.8 degrees and symptoms are reversed.
If not treated correctly, after two or more years often this becomes

4b. Irreversible clinical disease: The metabolic decline becomes increasingly irreversible, although mineral rebalancing will ease the effects, improve the metabolism, improve the circulation, improve the digestion, decrease the medication requirements, decrease the weight gain and slow the body's decline.

JC's Story

JC came to my office a little shyly. After all, I am a gynecologist, and, as a strapping young man, he clearly felt a little uneasy. What made me feel uncomfortable was not his gender, but the fact that he was carrying 254 pounds on his once 190-pound frame.

Although JC had not yet been diagnosed with type 2 diabetes, he was clearly insulin resistant and it seemed that a diagnosis of type 2 diabetes was an inevitable outcome of the metabolic failure that was creeping up on him. In fact, JC's father suffered from severe type 2 diabetes, and, at 300 pounds, he also had many other medical problems.

JC's HTMA showed significant calcium excess, sodium and potassium deficiency and thyroid hormone resistance nearly 10 times normal. His was a classic case of the Nutritional Disease Cascade. JC made no bones about it: he was frightened. He told me he was committed to making the necessary changes to bring his metabolism back into balance.

We began trace mineral supplementation, diet changes guided by the HTMA, which largely involved eliminating dietary calcium from dairy foods, and we added some supplements to help lower insulin resistance and correct his mineral imbalances.

His basal body temperatures confirmed what I expected based upon his HTMA results: a diagnosis of hypothyroidism (type 2) despite normal readings on his blood tests. This was causing his metabolism to slow considerably. He began taking Armour thyroid and gradually increased the dose to correct his metabolism while we were treating the underlying mineral imbalances.

He also began a daily walking program.

Over the next eight months, JC lost 60 pounds! He was energized and excited on the office visit that confirmed his relatively effortless weight loss. Gradually, we tapered off the thyroid medication and the nutritional supplements to maintenance doses.

JC has remained at his ideal body weight for a year now on a sensible diet that only restricts calcium intake and ensures he gets his ionic sea salt-derived minerals every day. Better yet, his blood sugars and insulin levels are normal! JC's almost inevitable diabetes was averted.

What a relief for both of us!

Metabolic failure

The thyroid hormone resistance and adrenal hormone resistance that leads to a slowed metabolic rate is a direct result of the Calcium Cascade from the intracellular calcium excess and sodium and potassium depletion. It's the inevitable result of sodium/potassium membrane electrical potential (S/PMEP) failure, which we discussed in detail in Chapter 4. Among other things, this sodium/potassium electrical energy differential across the cell membrane helps essential amino acids and glucose get into all the cells of our bodies—except fat cells, which use an entirely different process to absorb glucose independent of sodium.

Increased insulin levels due to insulin resistance actually stimulate the growth of fat cells. Fat cells absorb glucose without sodium, even if your body is severely sodium depleted. These cells are naturally stimulated to absorb increasing amounts of glucose by the increasing insulin levels, which directly further stimulates fat cells to grow larger and multiply.

When increased insulin levels are present, as in the case of insulin resistance (type 2 diabetes), weight gain is a huge problem in over 80 percent of our patients. We must treat and reverse this underlying insulin resistance and not just use medicines to increase insulin sensitivity. Fat cells in our bodies are a natural buffer mechanism for absorbing this excess glucose.

Insulin resistance leads to higher than normal release of insulin. Too much insulin causes blood sugars to drop after meals, leaving you feeling tired and sluggish and eventually this also leads to a low blood sugar roller coaster. The brain soon lacks glucose, its main "food," thereby stimulating your brain's appetite center to try to raise more glucose for your "starving" cells. The sugar or simple carb you recently ate has already turned to fat (stored energy) and this leads you to eat again to feel better quickly. These low blood sugars frequently lead to the misdiagnosis of "hypoglycemia" which is nothing more than a treatable early form of insulin resistance. If untreated, hypoglycemia will nearly always go on to develop into type 2 diabetes.

Unfortunately, fat cells can easily make more fat cells and take up greater amounts of our body's network of blood vessels, putting an increased workload on the heart and contributing to high blood pressure (hypertension). Fat cells continue to convert excess sugars into fat. Worse yet, since increased insulin levels prompt them to absorb more glucose, these fat cells continue to be stimulated to grow, thereby contributing to a vicious cycle of more insulin resistance and more weight gain, increased work for the heart and hypertension. Therefore, the use of insulin sensitizing drugs like metformin and rosiglitazone (Avandia) to treat the symptoms of increased blood sugar without treating and reversing the insulin resistance is not wise, and usually contributes to more rapid weight gain even with less caloric intake.

Drugs and weight loss are not the only answer. Treating the underlying mineral imbalance and the insulin resistance clearly can reverse this disease process and return the metabolism to normal, at least until this becomes an irreversible disease. I now have more than 100 type 2 diabetics in complete remission and they've achieved thousands of pounds of permanent weight loss and many more cases of type 2 diabetes prevented in my patients due to the correct treatment of the underlying malfunctioning metabolism and insulin resistance.

There are many effective diets and strategies for weight loss, but we must get off the weight roller coaster of lose, regain and relose. We must treat the underlying issues once and for all. Only this approach will achieve long-term success in treating and reversing weight issues.

The importance of treating the underlying problems of thyroid hormone resistance, insulin resistance and mineral imbalance can never be understated. We are getting fatter and fatter as a nation and it's getting worse. We should call your doctor's admonition to eat less and exercise more The Diet and Exercise Lie.

Your weight is of utmost importance to your long-term health. Stop the weight-loss roller coaster by paying attention to the underlying issues, most importantly insulin resistance, thyroid hormone resistance and mineral imbalances and deficiencies.

PART 2: FIVE TYPES OF HYPOTHYROIDISM

The thyroid, a tiny butterfly-shaped gland that straddles your windpipe and weighs less than an ounce, sends signals to every one of the trillions of cells in your body, billions of times every single day. It governs the metabolic rate of every cellular and bodily function. Without your thyroid, you'd wind down like a child's toy. Eventually, you would die.

Many experts believe that thyroid disease is the most underdiagnosed illness in America. We strongly agree. A paper published in the *Journal of the American Medical Association* nearly 60 years ago asserted that low thyroid function or hypothyroidism is the most common disease of those who enter a doctor's office—and it's the diagnosis doctors most often miss.

In my practice, I have found thyroid hormone resistance (as described for the first time in *The Calcium Lie* in 2008) is beyond epidemic level. It is now at a pandemic level and it is directly related to excess dietary calcium.

The problem is much worse today because most doctors will simply take a TSH (thyroid stimulating hormone) blood test and pronounce that your thyroid is "fine" based on outdated testing procedures and reference levels that are often "normal" even when you show all the classic signs of low thyroid function (hypothyroidism).

Physicians have so heavily relied on blood tests to make the diagnosis of hypothyroidism that they no longer recognize the actual symptoms and physical findings that often are present in patients with allegedly normal TSH levels that are actually clinically hypothyroid. That's why patients with the basket of low thyroid symptoms frequently have so much difficulty getting a diagnosis and treatment.

I estimate conservatively that 80 to 90 percent of the population has at least some degree of hypothyroidism. Clinical symptoms are present and yet patients' complaints are often unrecognized or ignored by doctors. In fact, many people with hypothyroidism have been labeled as hypochondriacs by one or more doctors and they are often treated for depression when their problem is actually low thyroid function.

Because hypothyroidism is so common, we're going to spend a fair amount of time with the subject and the easy ways you can address it and understand it. In short, all thyroid disease should be considered a disorder of production or a disorder of function, or some combination thereof, to make an accurate diagnosis. We will describe which type is which, but keep remembering, the symptoms are identical with all forms of the disease.

From the Calcium Cascade (Chapter 2), you already know that there is a connection between excess calcium, mineral deficiency and hypothyroidism. Before we go too far into this subject, I'd like to clearly define for the first time what I consider are the five different types of hypothyroidism:

Type 1 hypothyroidism is the failure of the thyroid glands to produce sufficient quantities of thyroid hormones to keep the body running properly. It is classically diagnosed by blood tests, specifically by a patient having an elevated TSH level (indicating low thyroid hormone production). The new upper level of "normal" was reduced to 3.0 by the American Endocrinology Association in 2011, but it should be much lower based on overwhelming scientific evidence. Most labs still report upper normal as around 4.5 (with a "normal" range of 0.45 to 4.5).

It has been shown that at least 30 percent of patients with a TSH above 2.0 have antithyroid antibodies that interfere with the production or action of the thyroid hormone. It has also been shown that pregnant women with TSH levels of 2.5 have a 15 percent increased miscarriage rate and another 15 percent increased risk for each point above 2.5. This 15 percent is added to the commonly observed average miscarriage rate of 15 percent, so a TSH of 2.5 equals a 30 percent rate of miscarriage, 3.5 equals 45 percent increased rate, 4.5 equals 60 percent increased rate. Note that most labs still rate a TSH of 4.5 as "upper normal."

Don't be fooled! These levels of TSH are not normal. The risk for virtually every disease associated with the aging process is increased if the TSH level is above 0.4. Most leading experts who truly understand hypothyroidism prefer a TSH level between 0.1 and 1.0.

Furthermore, there is no such thing as borderline hypothyroidism, only the failure to make a correct diagnosis. This type 1 form of hypothyroidism is associated with a failure of thyroid hormone production, which is probably in most cases related to chronic vitamin C deficiency, or alternatively bromine toxicity, L-tyrosine deficiency or low sodium levels and inability to get L-tyrosine into our thyroid cells or severe selenium deficiency.

The thyroid cannot make its hormone without the whole vitamin C molecule and ascorbic acid depletes this molecule from the body. (See Chapter 7.) This form of hypothyroidism (a failure of thyroid hormone production associated with increased TSH levels) is considered irreversible, and patients usually need to take supplemental hormone the rest of their lives. Unfortunately, it is diagnosed and treated incorrectly most of the time. (See type 5 below.)

Type 2 hypothyroidism is thyroid hormone resistance. Adequate levels of the hormones are being produced, but the body is simply not able to recognize or use them. Type 2 hypothyroidism is diagnosed by signs and symptoms, low basal body temperature (less than 97.8), and by ruling out type 1 hypothyroidism by having a more normal TSH of less than 2.0. The final diagnosis is confirmed by an abnormal intracellular calcium/potassium ratio on HTMA results with a ratio of these minerals inside the cells of the body of greater than 4.2:1.

These distinctions between type 1 and 2 hypothyroidism are very similar in principle to types 1 and 2 diabetes: type 1 diabetes being the failure of the pancreas to produce sufficient insulin to metabolize blood glucose (insulin deficiency), a disorder of production; type 2 diabetes being the body's inability to use the insulin that is being produced in sufficient or even excess quantities, i.e., insulin resistance.

Type 2 hypothyroidism should always be reversible by correcting or reversing the level of resistance as I've found again is also true in most cases of type 2 diabetes that have been diagnosed for less than two years.

It's common for people to have more than one type of thyroid disease. For example, patients with type 1 can still have thyroid hormone resistance, type 2, and they need slightly greater than normal hormone replacement doses to correct their metabolic rate.

Type 3 hypothyroidism is the presence of autoimmune thyroid disease, probably caused by bromine exposure or some other toxicity to the gland with secondary inflammation. It's usually called Hashimoto's thyroiditis, but there are several other forms, including chronic lymphocytic thyroiditis, Riedel's thyroiditis and chronic fibrous thyroiditis, all of which are associated with antithyroid gland or hormone antibodies.

The most common antibodies found on blood tests are the anti-thyroperoxidase antibody and anti-thyroglobulin antibody. In my experience, this illness seems to be reversible over time with correct supplementation and elimination of bromine from the body by giving enough iodine and sodium.

Like types 1 and 2 hypothyroidism, you can also have type 3 at the same time, further complicating matters. At least 30 percent of people with TSH levels above 2.0 have these abnormal antibodies and most of them have never had their antibodies tested before they came to me.

Low-dose cortisol may also be helpful in clearing the antibodies, according to the work of Dr. William Jeffries. Shark liver oil (not fish oil) also seems to make the antithyroid antibodies go away over time. Increasing iodine intake may also help, probably by helping eliminate the toxic bromine.

Type 4 hypothyroidism or severe selenium deficiency (SSD) is rare. I have seen only one case that I could actually accurately diagnose, but there may be many borderline cases and some type 1 patients may have severe selenium deficiency as an underlying cause of their problems.

It is diagnosed by reliable HTMA results confirming a severe selenium deficiency and basal body temperatures less than 97.8 degrees average. A critical factor when you're gathering the hair sample for the HTMA is that you have correctly followed the instructions and very precisely to eliminate the possibility of selenium contamination from hair products.

Type 5 hypothyroidism was described in 1992 by Dr. Denis Wilson as "Wilson's Temperature Syndrome." He associated the lower basal body temperatures and symptoms of hypothyroidism with an elevation of reverse T3 or RT3, a thyroid-blocking hormone of the actual active thyroid hormone called T3. Not surprisingly, the medical profession unfortunately ridiculed Wilson's observation, but he was definitely on the right track.

This form of the disease is actually caused by having an abnormal ratio of the total T3 thyroid hormones. Since T3 therapy stays in the body for only a short time, it is important to take thyroid hormones on an empty stomach two times a day, and never after dinner.

Most patients with type 5 hypothyroidism, if it is recognized at all, are merely being treated incorrectly with T4 alone (called Synthroid or levothyroxine). This is exactly how most of the people in the U.S. and worldwide are incorrectly treated for hypothyroidism today.

I suspect in the absence of T4 therapy alone as the cause, the most common underlying cause is that ever-present bromine interfering with iodine function and production of usable thyroid T3 hormones. Iodine supplementation has been shown to help reduce this.

This TT3/RT3 ratio test eliminates permanently the age-old dispute over treating hypothyroidism with T3 alone, T4 alone, or desiccated thyroid. The proof is in the test and the clinical correlation, which should be judged as complete correction of symptoms, correction of basal body temperatures to 97.8° or above, and metabolism being restored to normal.

This should be the goal of all treatments (irrespective of TSH levels), at least to the degree possible without changes in heart rate or palpitations or increased anxiousness. Various levels of sensitivity to therapy occur and require individualized treatment. In general, gradual increases are safer with monthly assessments of basal body temperatures (BBT) and most importantly, the resting heart rate.

Editor's Note to Readers

These descriptions of the types of hypothyroidism are Dr. Thompson's discoveries, based on his 13 years of clinical experience with patients with these conditions and his wide knowledge of biochemistry, physiology and human nutrition. The medical profession does not generally recognize them thus far, and, in fact, they are being described as five distinct types in this book for the first time. It would not be surprising if they are ridiculed by mainstream medical practitioners out of ignorance.

Knowing your HTMA level of thyroid hormone resistance, blood tests for TT3/RT3 ratios and basal body temperatures (for all five types of the disease) corrected to 97.8 remain the acid tests for the correct treatment of this disease.

This makes it highly unlikely you will find a doctor who is well versed in the diagnosis and treatment of types 1 to 5 hypothyroidism, unless he/she has read this book.

Dr. Thompson would be happy to consult with your doctor on your case provided the correct information is available. Contact him through his office at 907-260-6914.

Is hypothyroidism your problem?

Here's a laundry list of the most common symptoms of all types of hypothyroidism. Keep in mind that this is not definitive since other conditions, especially adrenal problems, can cause the same symptoms.

The symptoms will be the same with every type of hypothyroidism, so laboratory testing and HTMA testing results, along with reliable basal body temperature (BBT) measurements, are all essential to accurately determine the type of hypothyroidism, and how to treat patients correctly. If you have more than two of these symptoms and BBTs below 97.8 for three days in a row of taking your temperature first thing in the morning before you get out of bed, it's worth investigating the possibility you have low thyroid hormone levels or function.

Hypothyroid Symptoms

- Obesity
- Inappropriate weight gain
- Difficulty losing weight
- Fatigue, lethargy, midafternoon energy loss, sleepiness
- Depression
- Constipation
- Restlessness
- Mood swings
- Difficulty concentrating, memory impairment
- Cold hands and feet, cold intolerance
- Basal body temperatures (BBT) below 97.8 degrees
- Coarse, dry hair
- Hair falling out, brittle nails, baldness
- Skin coarse, dry, scaly and thick, especially on elbows, heels and feet
- Decreased perspiration
- Dry mouth and eyes and/or diagnosis of Sjogren's Syndrome
- Hoarse or gravelly voice, slowed speech

- Acne
- Puffiness and swelling around eyes and face, wrists or ankles
- Aches and pains in joints, hands and feet
- Fibromyalgia, muscle cramps and weakness, muscle pain, numbness
- Arthritis, gout
- Carpal tunnel syndrome, tarsal tunnel syndrome (feet)
- Irregular menstrual cycles, ovarian cysts, fibrocystic breasts, PMS
- Low sex drive
- Frequent infections, especially skin problems
- Snoring/sleep apnea
- Shortness of breath and tightness in chest
- Tinnitus (ringing in ears)
- Thinning or complete absence of outer third of eyebrows
- Headaches, hypertension, hyporeflexia (diminished reflexes)
- Goiter or gland atrophy

- Growth failure and delay, short stature
- Jaundice in newborn

- Enlarged tongue, difficulty swallowing
- Loss of sense of smell and taste

Hypothyroidism is incredibly simple to diagnose, but those who suffer from this debilitating condition often spend years looking for a doctor who will confirm the obvious diagnosis. That's because modern medicine has become so fixated on blood tests with falsely expanded normal values instead of good patient care and reliable patient histories. Most doctors today have become lax about physical exams and actually taking a good history and spending enough time to carefully look at a patient. Lab tests, HTMA and basal body temperature data are essential, but the physician who conducts them is extremely rare.

Unfortunately for many patients, blood tests often complicate matters leading to under- or misdiagnosis of the disease. All too often, blood tests lead to a denial of treatment of many people who need it because of the ignorance of doctors practicing a seriously flawed belief system that relies on TSH alone, incorrectly interpreted laboratory tests and T4 therapy alone in the treatment of documented hypothyroidism

Basal Body Temperature

Here's how to diagnose basic hypothyroidism with nearly 100 percent certainty. You can do it yourself. If you're a woman and still menstruating, do this in the first ten days of your cycle, day 1 being the day your period starts.

Get yourself a good oral thermometer (digital is easiest; I recommend the Timex® brand, which takes only 6 seconds). Put it by your bed when you retire for the night. First thing in the morning, before you get out of bed or move around much, take your temperature orally. If your average temperature is 97.8 degrees Fahrenheit (36.5 degrees Celsius) or less for three consecutive days, it is almost certain your thyroid function is low and your metabolism is slowed.

You need laboratory tests and an HTMA test with a reliable calcium/potassium ratio to make an accurate diagnosis. To tell if your thermometer is working correctly, check your temperature twice in a row, any time. If the digital thermometer is off by more than 0.1 degrees on repeat testing, replace it. Accuracy is critical.

Getting a diagnosis

Over the past 40 years or more, the American Endocrinology Association and independent laboratories have continued to expand the "normal" ranges of TSH (thyroid stimulating hormone, a commonly used marker to determine if a person has low thyroid function) precisely because so much of our population s affected with impaired thyroid hormone function. Laboratories are required to continually readjust their normal values like a bell curve in school. Only a certain percentage is allowed to be reported as abnormal. As the population becomes increasingly abnormal in terms of thyroid hormone production or resistance, the reported number of abnormals has to stay the same, causing a severe underreporting of this increasingly common disease.

Type 1 Hypothyroidism

Basal body temperatures (BBTs) were the gold standard for diagnosing hypothyroidism for more than 50 years before blood tests first became available in the early 1970s. BBTs below 97.8 degrees Fahrenheit (36.5 Celsius) were considered necessary for the accurate diagnosis of hypothyroidism. Since these blood tests became available, the TSH elevation has become the most common criteria for a diagnosis of type 1 hypothyroidism (above 3.0, American Endocrinology Association's newly established reference range in 2011). The current trend is to consider 0.1 to 1.0 the ideal normal TSH level, but I'm not sure the TSH matters once an accurate clinical diagnosis is made. Certainly, if your basal body temperature is still low and the baseline resting heart rate is unchanged, then you are definitely not being overtreated regardless of the TSH level. Total T3 may be the most important diagnostic tool.

Type 2 Hypothyroidism

Type 2 hypothyroidism or thyroid hormone resistance is caused by an intracellular calcium/potassium imbalance in all the cells of the body, caused by far too much calcium and far too little potassium inside these cells, neutralizing the effects of the thyroid hormones that are produced, and making them ineffective in governing our bodies' metabolic functions.

For people with type 2 hypothyroidism, thyroid hormone blood tests may be normal, so doctors won't recognize this syndrome unless they do a hair tissue mineral analysis (HTMA) from a reliable lab that is correctly reporting the all-important intracellular calcium/potassium ratios, plus a careful symptom review and case history. A reliable oral basal body temperature must be measured at least three days each month, before ovulation in menstruating women as noted earlier.

In reviewing my records for the past seven years, I have found more than 95 percent correlation between a HTMA result showing an elevated ratio of calcium to potassium and low basal body temperatures. This confirms that the intracellular calcium/potassium imbalance causes type 2 hypothyroidism, thyroid hormone resistance.

HTMA test results should be a part of the diagnosis and treatment of everyone with hypothyroidism since type 2 disease has become so common. If you are currently being treated with T4 (Synthroid or levothyroxine) alone for type 1 hypothyroidism, you will have a very low TT3/RT3 ratio and will in most cases remain clinically hypothyroid no matter what the TSH level. Correct treatment must therefore include adequate T3 replacement (Cytomel or liothyronine) along with the T4. Due to the short half-life of T3, it must be given two times per day (upon awakening, on an empty stomach and no food for at least 30 minutes and a second dose 6 to 8 hours later). T4 (levothyroxine) can still be one time per day, without food, taken first thing upon waking.

Virtually every one of my patients who has a low basal body temperature with an elevated calcium/potassium ratio (type 2 resistance-type hypothyroidism) is put on supplemental thyroid hormones. This form of hypothyroidism is reversible over time by correcting the intracellular calcium and potassium levels and the ratio. In order to make this correction, it is important to make specific diet changes according to your HTMA results. Also, specific supplements may be recommended. In addition to this, I frequently use a medication called spironolactone (or Aldactone), which helps decrease the urinary potassium loss thereby meaningfully shortening the length of time it takes to correct the calcium/potassium ratio.

Without exception, you'll get better over time and feel better right away or as soon as the correct dosages are achieved. Your energy will improve, skin conditions will often resolve, and hair and nails will grow strong and healthy again. As your basal body temperatures improve, you'll warm up, depression and mood often improve and, among other things, you'll lose weight.

What's more, by showing patients their HTMA results, and by giving them specific dietary and supplement recommendations, we begin to reverse the underlying disease process and eventually eliminate the need for the thyroid medication. That's correct. Type 2 Hypothyroidism is reversible and so are types 3, 4, and 5 in my experience. I encourage patients to give up their calcium supplements and dairy products and take ionic mineral supplements to restore their mineral levels and balance. What could be simpler?

I have treated nearly 2,000 patients over the past 13 years with the incorporation of HTMA results into their care. With the inclusion of the HTMA results in patient's treatment and diet recommendations, the patient's success in improving their health is amazing. Treating and often reversing the underlying medical problems nutritionally with the best scientific accuracy possible and preventing even more health problems with the incorporation of the HTMA results into their care is truly a rewarding endeavor for me and my patients. I often remind my patients that their success is also my success. That partnership requires accountability on both sides of the equation.

Most importantly, this treatment plan works in every compliant patient. Unfortunately, finances are a limitation for most people and insurance and Medicare will not pay for nutritional supplements. This makes it even more important to make recommendations that are reliable, scientifically valid and reproducible. I know without a doubt, this is absolutely true for HTMA results and the nutritional recommendations in this book. I have proven it time and again in my practice.

If you are hypothyroid, as diagnosed by low basal body temperature, you'll need thyroid hormone replacement and ionic mineral supplements, plus some dietary changes that will almost certainly include eliminating dairy products, high-calcium cruciferous vegetables like broccoli, cabbage, kale, and cauliflower and increases of potassium-rich foods like asparagus, peas, beans, beets, celery, oranges, dates, plums, raisins, cantaloupe and, in some cases, bananas.

We'll warn you: Your return to health won't be instantaneous. It may take several years or more to begin to get your mineral levels back into balance and rein in the calcium excess, but you'll feel better and better every day along the way.

A word of caution: Look for the mineral supplement product that has my name on the label. Other similar-looking products are not correctly formulated.

In my experience with reliable HTMA testing over the past 13 years, it is clear that this one single test has had a greater impact on my patients' health in the short and long term than any other lab test known to medical science. The HTMA test has the potential to bring science to nutrition and rational thought to healthcare practitioners who choose to help their patients get better health.

Mainstream medicine's bulldog-like determination to diagnose hypo-thyroidism based on only one criterion, the TSH, has led to The Thyroid Stimulating Hormone Lie, which has left millions to suffer needlessly.

In summary, "acceptable" laboratory TSH levels have continued to rise at least in part because thyroid hormone production and function is impaired from various nutritional shortfalls and imbalances, including:

• Trace mineral deficiencies

• Deficiency of whole-food vitamin C complex (as whole-food, not ascorbic acid, which causes C deficiency, leading to thyroid hormone production failure)

• Sodium and potassium deficiency (leading to thyroid hormone resistance)

• Selenium deficiency (leading to thyroid hormone production failure)

• Amino acid deficiencies (associated with intracellular low sodium, especially tyrosine, leading to thyroid hormone production failure)

• Monosaccharide deficiencies for building protein receptors, potentially leading to the development of antithyroid antibodies and bromine toxicity

TSH levels above 0.4 (the lowest level that is considered normal) have been associated with increased risk of thyroid cancer, increased weight, increased breast and prostate cancer risk, abnormal lipid profiles, increased insulin resistance, hypertension, autoimmune thyroid disease, increased risk of cardiovascular disease, increased depression, as well as clinically significant hypothyroidism. (References courtesy Dr. Thierry Hertoghe.) Please seek help if your BBTs are below 97.8. TSH levels are only helpful in making a diagnosis of type 1 hypothyroidism.

PART 3: INSULIN RESISTANCE

We skimmed the topic of insulin resistance and its effects on your weight earlier in this chapter. But you might have already guessed there's more.

Insulin resistance, whether it manifests as obesity, type 2 diabetes or as some sort of "pre-diabetes" often called metabolic syndrome, means blood sugar metabolism is impaired because of insulin resistance. Insulin resistance now affects 1 in 4 Americans or about 68 million people.

In the coming decades, this horrifying statistic will play havoc with our health as a nation, not only in the physical sense, but also in lost productivity and skyrocketing medical costs that are already in the stratosphere. It is estimated at the current rate of increase, by the year 2030 nearly 95 percent of adults in the U.S. will have some form of insulin resistance.

Insulin resistance has few, if any symptoms. Most people have no idea they have it. However, people with chronic hypoglycemia (low blood sugar) and those who are overweight already have significant insulin resistance. These people are merely overcompensating for the blood sugar drops (called hypoglycemia) by eating more sugar, setting up a cycle of sugar highs and lows and interim hyperinsulin releases leading to weight gain.

Insulin resistance is most often a nutritional deficiency disease, not a hereditary familial illness as we have been brainwashed to believe. It is our eating habits, and therefore our resulting mineral deficiencies and imbalances, that run in families due to similar food likes and dislikes and cultural and locality dietary habits that lead to the problem.

I refer to this as The Familial Disease Lie. These family eating habits are the most common pathway to all nutritional deficiency- and imbalance-related disease. We grow up learning to like certain foods. We buy what we like repeatedly from the store and thereby end up with similar family mineral deficiencies and imbalances leading to many of our health problems. Having the HTMA results helps us to see accurately what is going on and leads to meaningful long-term changes of these levels and imbalances through scientifically accurate diet and supplement changes.

If you typically get very tired, cranky or ravenously hungry if a mealtime passes without food, you may have insulin resistance.

Here are the most common symptoms of type 2 diabetes:

- Extreme thirst
- Excessive urination
- Hunger
- Unintentional weight loss
- Easy weight gain and difficult loss

- Fatigue
- Irritability
- Slow wound healing
- Blurred vision
- Tingling or numbness in feet
- Recurrent infections

How do you know if you have insulin resistance? In type 2 (insulin-resistant) diabetes, large amounts of "free" insulin circulate through the body, since the cells are unable to use it to balance blood sugars. Since insulin belongs in your cells, excessive amounts of insulin circulating through your bloodstream in proportion to blood sugar levels taken at the same time are the best indicators for diagnosing insulin resistance. This test is called the glucose to insulin or G/I ratio.

Always ask your doctor to test your blood insulin level, along with your glucose level, to determine your G/I ratio. These two tests must be done simultaneously to be meaningful. A low ratio, especially one below 7, is very abnormal in my experience and suggests significant insulin resistance.

Here's something very important: If you are obese, you almost certainly have some degree of insulin resistance. Many authorities now say fasting blood glucose above 90 is abnormal and should be considered an early sign of increasing insulin resistance. Current medical practice is to use a blood sugar reading of 100–124 as borderline diabetes. Taking enough Chrome-Mate (chromium polynicotinate) will almost always reverse this problem in the first two years, after which the resistance may become less reversible.

When most doctors test for diabetes, they check blood glucose levels alone, not insulin levels. The beauty of knowing your insulin level (or more specifically the G/I ratio) is that it can help you diagnose and begin treating insulin resistance long before it actually becomes type 2 diabetes. I also consider triglyceride levels of over 100 and fasting insulin levels of over 10 signs of significant insulin resistance.

You've no doubt heard that type 2 diabetes is not curable. You've heard of the multitude of expensive drugs used to treat it. You've also probably heard that the risk of heart disease in diabetics is high and that it actually kills 2 out of 3 diabetics, not to speak of the increased risk of kidney failure, blindness and peripheral neuropathy that leads to impaired wound healing and necessitates more amputations than accidents cause.

Insulin resistance is part of the Calcium Cascade we described earlier. (You might want to review it.) When excess calcium and mineral shortfalls combine with amino acid deficiencies, they lead to the failure of the sodium/potassium membrane electrical potential S/PMEP, the body's only means of getting essential amino acids and glucose into all of your cells, except fat cells. These cells (except fat cells) become starved for glucose and trigger cravings for more and more sugary and salty foods, setting up another vicious cycle of craving for more sugar, leading to more insulin resistance as more insulin is needed to help normalize blood glucose levels. The absorption of the excess glucose into fat cells, stimulated by the increased insulin levels, leads to wildly reproducing and rapidly growing fat cells. It's a downhill slide. Please hear us say once more, it is time to get off this weight roller coaster once and for all by treating and reversing the underlying insulin resistance.

What mainstream medicine fails to recognize is that the insulin receptors that live on the outer lining of those cells can be regenerated over time in most patients through proper nutrition and supplementation, thereby reversing most type 2 diabetes.

At the risk of sounding like a broken record, you know what that means: Increase your intake of sodium through easily absorbable natural sea salt, rock salts, ionic mineral supplements and chromium polynicotinate (not the cheaper picolinate form, proven not to work or work as well) should be taken with every meal (sold as ChromeMate under many brand names, also referred to as "GTF" Chromium). This combination will resupply the body with the correct form of the essential amino acids, nicotinic acid, and chromium needed to redevelop insulin receptors. Vitamin C in its whole-food form (not as ascorbic acid) and vitamin B3 in its whole-food form (as richly found in stabilized rice bran) are also needed to help this change occur.

I have personally treated more than 100 patients with clinically diagnosed type 2 diabetes of less than two years duration. In over 95 percent of the cases, where the patient was compliant with diet and supplement changes, the diabetes was completely reversed. That means blood sugars remain normal without medication. That's something that rarely happens in the medical world. That's why I'm so sure I am on the right track in terms of treating and reversing the underlying cause of insulin resistance and the accurate treatment of type 2 diabetes.

I find that any patient can do this, not by particularly rigorous diet, weight loss, and exercise regimens, which are most commonly recommended by the medical profession (although these don't hurt), but by starting the correct mineral replacement, correcting important mineral ratios, whole-food vitamin C and supplementation with the right form of chromium with every meal, and by taking enough and sticking with it.

In my experience, ChromeMate nearly always works to reduce insulin resistance and weight if it is taken with every meal and if enough is taken. It is even more effective if also taken at bedtime. I use 600 mcg capsules only because 200 mcg doses are inconvenient and more expensive. There is no known human toxicity of this type of chromium in humans at any level. The dose needed clearly depends on the level or resistance.

What is amazing is that, over time with adequate and correct Chrome-Mate intake, the blood glucose levels remain normal and steady, even if you miss taking the whole-food supplements now and then. Weight returns to normal, energy and healing improve, and cancer, heart disease, vascular disease and dementia risk are significantly reduced. Insulin levels decline to normal, hemoglobin A1C returns to normal (below 5.6), and G/I ratios increase, over time. I call this remission. Once remission is achieved for over 6 to 24 months, less ChromeMate is needed to maintain it.

All weight-loss regimens, no matter what form, without treating the underlying metabolism (thyroid hormone resistance), mineral imbalances and insulin resistance, will be met with eventual failure. Get off the weight roller coaster and stay off by treating the underlying problem. Even if medications are needed, they should be temporary.

PART 4: ADRENAL INSUFFICIENCY/SUPPRESSION

Your adrenal glands, two walnut-sized glands that sit on top of your kidneys, produce hormones that help control heart rate and blood pressure, fight infection, respond to stress, regulate the way your body uses food and many other vital functions. More importantly, the adrenals produce natural steroids that regulate mineral levels in your blood, especially magnesium, sodium and potassium.

No doubt you can see where this is going.

If your body has a calcium excess, the adrenal glands are reducing their function, or their ability to produce adrenal gland hormones is being suppressed in order for the body to retain the necessary magnesium, to attempt to balance the high calcium levels. This is a normal body response gone awry. When the adrenal hormones called mineralocorticoids are suppressed, sodium and potassium are continually lost in the urine and your body becomes deficient in these critical minerals.

Symptoms of adrenal insufficiency, suppression, exhaustion, resistance, and impending failure can include the following symptoms:

- Headache
- Profound weakness
- Fatigue
- Dry skin
- Slow, sluggish movement
- Loss of appetite
- Unintentional weight loss
- Joint pain
- Abdominal pain
- Nausea
- Vomiting
- Dehydration
- Unusual and excessive sweating on face and/or palms

- Low blood pressure (orthostatic, drops with standing up more than normal)
- Skin rash or lesions
- High fever
- Shaking chills
- Confusion or coma
- Darkening of the skin
- Rapid heart rate
- Rapid breathing
- Flank pain
- Decreased resistance to infection and cancer
- Constipation
- Increased allergies

I find it fascinating that adrenal deficiency symptoms are basically identical to the constellation of symptoms associated with the flu (caused by the influenza virus). The reason for this is also enlightening and a great way to help us remember the adrenal deficiency symptoms. The influenza virus has figured out how to mimic our hypothalamic-releasing factor for adrenal cortisol production, thus turning off the pituitary adrenal stimulating hormones, suppressing adrenal cortisol production.

It is this "mimicry" at the hypothalamic level in the brain that leads to suppression of cortisol production with the resulting sudden adrenal "flu" symptoms. The degree of virulence of a particular strain of the flu virus depends on the quality or accuracy of the likeness or the degree of mimicry of the amino acid sequences of the particular strain of the virus with our body's own hypothalamic-releasing hormone amino acid sequences.

Normally, when any infection is starting, our bodies release cortisol at 4 to 10 times the normal levels for the first 48 to 72 hours of the illness to jazz up the immune system to fight the virus or infection. The lack of this release leads to immune compromise. What a smart virus this is! This is why for many years, pediatric doctors routinely gave IV cortisol to children in the initial treatment of severe life threatening infections (a practice that is less common today unfortunately, except in pediatricians still practicing who were trained in the '60s or early '70s).

It's also interesting to note that many of the symptoms of adrenal fatigue are identical to the symptoms of hypothyroidism. You've probably already figured out that there is a close relationship there.

Since most people today believe The Sodium Lie, that they should reduce salt intake to avoid high blood pressure, they become progressively even more sodium and iodine depleted. The sodium is sucked out of their cells to make up for the deficiency. The continuous loss of sodium from our cells eventually leads to failure of the sodium/potassium membrane electrical potential and inability to get amino acids and glucose into our cells (except fat cells), inability to produce stomach acid correctly and poor protein digestion, as we discussed at length in Chapter 4.

Increasing adrenal hormone suppression due to excess calcium leads to:

• Further slowing of the metabolism;

• Inability to cope with stress;

• Adrenal exhaustion from release of increasing amounts of adrenal hormones to try to compensate;

• Lack of sufficient energy production;

• Various mineral and vitamin deficiencies;

- Decreased or diminished immune responses;

- Increased problems with allergies;

- Increased cancer risk;

- Increased and more severe infections, especially viral illnesses, and more.

I speculate that the increased cancer and medical problems related to "vitamin" D hormone deficiency are more likely related to D hormone suppression from intracellular calcium excess thus leading to adrenal suppression with a resulting increase in illnesses. Nevertheless, as we note in Chapter 7, I still correct D hormone levels to around 40–60, to be sure this hormone is not deficient. Higher D hormone levels in people who already have an intracellular calcium excess will lead to more of all the calcium excess problems we describe in this book.

Adrenal malfunction can have long-reaching emotional consequences, including anxiety, withdrawal and indecision, and physical ones as well, including increasing numbers and severity of infections, more frequent viral illnesses and increased cancer risk. Most adrenal issues can be corrected merely by using more sea salt, especially when you and your doctor know through an HTMA that your intracellular sodium level is low.

How do you know if you have adrenal malfunction?

Adrenal insufficiency or suppression is much more common than conventional medicine acknowledges, and it often goes hand-in-hand with the other metabolic malfunction, insulin resistance and thyroid hormone resistance, autoimmune disease, allergies and chronic illness.

Tissue mineral analysis for calcium/potassium and sodium/magnesium ratios and thyroid function tests along with basal body temperatures are as useful in establishing a diagnosis of adrenal insufficiency as is a history of recurring illnesses such as acquiring common colds easily, having somewhat prolonged illnesses, or any autoimmune or chronic illness such as rheumatoid arthritis. Adrenal hormone levels may also be measured accurately with saliva and urine testing. However, if reserves are low, this testing may still be fairly normal.

In HTMA testing, the minerals most often linked with adrenal hormone function are sodium and magnesium. The correct ratio of sodium to magnesium has been established to be 4.0. Therefore, if a patient has a ratio of 1.0, the patient would be expected to be four times below normal in adrenal hormone response or adrenal hormone function.

CAT scans or MRIs may actually show calcium deposits in the adrenal glands. That's an interesting confirmation of the problems of excess calcium.

I treat adrenal insufficiency or suppression with increased amounts of sodium to help reawaken and correct the S/PMEP and help restore the digestion of proteins carrying the essential amino acids that are needed to help restore the adrenal hormone levels, function and the mineral balance. Of course, I also use sea salt and balanced ionic trace minerals, and I frequently add supplements like DHEA, taurine, tyrosine, iodine, copper, vitamin C complex (not ascorbic acid—see Chapter 7), methyl-donors like MSM and, in some cases, low-dose bioidentical cortisol.

POINTS TO REMEMBER

✔ In the midst of unparalleled food wealth and unprecedented obesity, we as a nation are literally starving for the minerals we need in the proper balance so our bodies can function properly. These mineral deficiencies and imbalances lead to food cravings, salt cravings and numerous negative metabolic changes.

✔ Rebalancing minerals and reducing insulin resistance effectively treats obesity and changes metabolism over time, stopping the weight gain-loss-gain roller coaster.

✔ Metabolic failure is associated with hypothyroidism, insulin resistance and adrenal suppression. All of these are downstream results of the failure of the sodium/potassium membrane electrical potential and intracellular calcium excess. When mineral deficiencies exist, especially low sodium and potassium, which are the most common, this membrane failure and poor stomach acid production lead to poor protein digestion, reduced absorption of amino acids and a host of metabolic imbalances. These metabolic issues can be corrected in most cases with proper supplementation, specific nutritional changes and rebalancing the body's mineral levels when based on reliable HTMA results.

✔ All types of hypothyroidism can be definitively diagnosed by a simple basal body temperature test, indicating slowed metabolic rate. If your body temperatures on awakening are consistently low, less than or equal to 97.8 degrees Fahrenheit, treatment with thyroid hormones will almost always produce positive results. Thyroid hormone resistance, or more specifically type 2 is caused by an abnormal intracellular calcium/potassium ratio. It is measurable, reproducible and can accurately predict the degree of thyroid hormone resistance, and the temporary need for thyroid hormone replacement. Correcting the calcium/potassium ratio also reverses the disease.

✔ Type 2 diabetes can almost always be treated with mineral and nutritional supplementation and can most often be reversed in the early stages when treated correctly.

✔ Adrenal insufficiency is often diagnosed by excess calcium in the blood or calcium deposits in the adrenal glands themselves. Determining the sodium/magnesium ratio from the HTMA specifically reveals the degree of adrenal hormone resistance or reduced ability of this hormone to do its work. Salivary hormone levels or 24-hour urine hormone levels can also help show adrenal hormone deficiencies or suppression. Increasing sodium and potassium intake to reawaken the sodium/potassium membrane electrical potential and adding other specific HTMA-directed supplements and, in some cases, low-dose cortisol hormone supplementation, in addition to dietary changes will almost always reverse the condition over time.

CHAPTER 6

Women's Issues: Pregnancy, Childbirth and Menopause

By training and board certification, I am a gynecologist and obstetrician or an ob-gyn in the lingo. I admit I'm a little mushy when it comes to pregnant ladies and babies. I love them! In more than 30 years of nurturing women through their pregnancies and catching their babies, I have learned wonderful ways to help women stay healthy throughout their pregnancies and to deliver healthy babies.

It breaks my heart to see the lack of nutritional guidance our pregnant patients get from conventional doctors and lack of nutritional leadership in the profession. Maybe there are just too many commercial interests out there competing at the expense of our patients. I have to believe that this lack of proper care comes from ignorance on the part of their doctors (I suffered from it too, for many years), from lack of nutrition training, intellectual laziness and a propensity to believe the status quo, with an indoctrinated dependence on drugs or surgery to treat everything. All of that is combined with the unfortunate amnesia about the biochemistry courses that accompany all doctors' medical training.

The truth is that when women become pregnant, in most cases they become hypervigilant about their health, since that health directly affects their babies. I can say without doubt that this is a medical message that has "gotten through" and this one is to their benefit and that of their unborn children. While this attention to our health should be in place throughout our lives and, for women, it should be especially a concern when you are planning a pregnancy, we'll take what we can get.

If you are pregnant or planning a pregnancy, please pay attention here. This chapter has information vital to your health and your baby's well-being.

Bear with us. We don't mean to be insulting here, but this is important.

Human beings are animals. In fact, we are mammals and all mammals have similar physiology.

While I don't agree with much that Joel Wallach says in his 1996 book *Dead Doctors Don't Lie*, Wallach was right on target when he noted that farmers have known for more than 50 years that their animals need sea salt (or rock salt) in order to remain healthy and to breed without birth defects. Wallach is a veterinarian, not a doctor or a biochemist, which is why he is so wrong about so many things he espouses, especially the use of colloidal minerals, but he's right about salt.

Yet there is a ring of truth in much of what Wallach says when he proposes that humans can achieve their maximum biological life span through proper nutrition and an adequate supply of vitamins and minerals. To attain a long life, he advises people to take charge of their own health rather than rely on the advice of their physicians, who, in his view, make poor role models in terms of their own health and longevity.

As a boy who grew up on a cattle ranch and studied animal husbandry in college, Wallach knows his stuff about rock salt on the farm.

He writes, "What's the first thing a farmer or a rancher puts out for his livestock? A big salt block, right? Nobody gives any restriction on a cow, she goes out and has all the salt that she wants."

Any farmer worth his salt (pardon the pun) knows that unrefined sea salt is essential to the health of his animals and to his livelihood. Wallach talks in great depth about the increased incidence of birth defects on farms where animals do not have free access to salt. He concludes rock salt has eliminated 98 percent of birth defects and 70 percent of miscarriages in farm animal breeding. Lack of salt is synonymous with increased risk of birth defects, miscarriage, organ failure, premature aging and death at a young age.

Salt is so essential to the health of mammals that wild elephants will risk their lives to get to the salt licks in remote caves.

Why do mammals need salt? If you've been paying attention to the first five chapters, you already know the answer: Natural unrefined sea salt or rock salt from ancient sea beds, the correct type used on most farms, contains all of the minerals we need for survival, in perfect proportions. That applies to humans just as well as to farm animals.

In the biological sense, our cells are no different from those of farm animals and wild elephants in their basic biochemistry. We need our salt and *all* of the minerals it contains, not just iodine or sodium or chloride or calcium. Yes, sea salt is naturally iodized. If the label says iodine is added, they are lying to you. If the sea salt does not contain iodine, it is not sea salt or it has been processed. We need real sea salt.

When you're pregnant

Now think about what happens in a woman's body when she becomes pregnant. She has a little life growing inside her and it has its needs. That baby will get its needs fulfilled as much as possible, no matter what.

Let's say that the average woman weighs 150 pounds. We know that the human body is approximately 72 percent water and 28 percent minerals. Extrapolating that to body weight, that means she is carrying around 42 pounds of minerals—or she should be, if she is completely healthy.

As the baby grows, it draws minerals from Mom's body. Over the course of a 265-day pregnancy, the baby takes about four pounds of minerals from the mother or about 10 percent of her total mineral supply.

Now, babies are not parasites. Biologically they are called saprophytes. This means that, by perhaps some law of survival of future generations, babies get what they want and need, at the expense of the mother's health if necessary, even *in utero*. So if the baby needs a mineral that is in short supply in the mother's body, the baby will take it anyway, leaving Mom even shorter on some essential minerals than before pregnancy. On the other hand, if the mother has an excess of a mineral, for example calcium or copper, that excess will be passed on to the baby as a mineral fingerprint of the mother. This is obviously by design for babies to be born with as near a perfect mineral balance as possible.

Every pregnant woman needs major mineral replacement through a high-quality ionic mineral supplement in quantities to bring her mineral levels up to normal before pregnancy and to replace those that are inevitably lost through pregnancy, childbirth and breast-feeding.

In my experience, we all need about 3 grams of ionic trace sea salt derived minerals daily to meet our daily loss. This is about 6 tablets or $1^1/_2$ tsp of the liquid trace minerals daily. If we merely divide the loss of 4 pounds of minerals to the baby over the 265 days of the pregnancy, at 300 tablets per 8-ounce container, then each mother needs to take at least 15 tablets or at least 7.5 grams per day of trace minerals to stay "even" with respect to her overall mineral loss through the end of the pregnancy. If deficiency is already present, which is almost always the case, more minerals may be helpful and important.

Mineral intake is a very close second place to water as the most important supplement pregnant women should be taking during pregnancy. Almost no pregnant women are getting the minerals they need, except my patients. The imbalanced and inadequate chelated minerals in our current prenatal "vitamins" (which are drugs, not vitamins) are quite literally woefully inadequate and may actually be harmful.

A woman pays a price for every pregnancy. Pregnancies that are too close together take an even bigger toll. One of the earliest signs of mineral depletion is dental cavities and broken teeth. I always ask my patients about their teeth and they usually seem a little surprised at the question. A recent rash of cavities is a surefire sign that the woman is severely minerally depleted.

Think back to Chapters 2 and 3. Bones are made of at least 12 different minerals. Bones and teeth have generally the same basic mineral composition, so signs of a breakdown in the teeth are also signs of mineral deficiency. Listen up, dentists: You can help resolve this problem too! Also, periodontal disease is largely contributed to by vitamin C deficiency in part caused by ascorbic acid, which depletes vitamin C.

When we start looking at the impact of a number of illnesses that commonly affect pregnancy including hypertension, preeclampsia, gestational diabetes, hemorrhage, placental abruption and excess weight gain, it becomes clear that these problems are nearly all related to nutritional deficiencies and imbalances that are totally preventable and treatable with taking the correct supplements and minerals. The same is true for conditions so prevalent after pregnancy, including depression, anxiety, weight gain, hypothyroidism and more.

Conventional medicine seems to agree that pregnant women need supplements, so a prescription prenatal "vitamin" supplement is provided that is little more than calcium, iron and folic acid, a B vitamin (folate) known to help prevent one type of birth defect and a few other drug-form "vitamins." (More about birth defects later.) Now, conventional medicine is telling pregnant women that they need calcium to keep their bone density during pregnancy when the baby is drawing on the mother's mineral supply. Duh! It's the *mineral* supply, not the calcium supply that moms need. See, you're already smarter than your doctor!

Mothers need a complete mineral supplement that they can absorb and use, not just calcium! Patients often tell me their "vitamins" have minerals. Unfortunately, very few supplements have the right minerals or the right kind of minerals. They may even have the wrong minerals or minerals that are not needed or can even be harmful. However, if the woman doesn't know her exact needs from a reliable HTMA test, she may be making a big mistake when she chooses her supplements. Every pregnant woman and her doctor need to know for sure. (More about the "vitamins" in Chapter 7.)

The mineral drawdown during pregnancy can cause a host of post-pregnancy problems. What woman hasn't struggled with shedding excess poundage acquired during the pregnancy? Many suffer from postpartum depression. And down the road a few years, 70 percent of the women who had gestational diabetes will develop type 2 diabetes without the interventions covered in Chapter 5.

For the most part, conventional medicine only uses drugs to deal with these problems during pregnancy and afterward. You've read far enough in this book now to know that type 2 diabetes, type 2 hypothyroidism, obesity, migraine headaches, insomnia, anxiety and depression are all related to mineral status and that correcting these mineral deficiencies and imbalances will treat, reverse and prevent these diseases.

It's worth a few paragraphs here to discuss gestational diabetes, since it is such a serious and increasingly common problem in pregnancy that leads to even more serious problems years later in over 70 percent of patients.

Doctors fail to diagnose at least 20 percent of today's cases of gestational diabetes because they have failed to consider the significance of the insulin resistance measurement in accurately diagnosing the problem. Unfortunately, when they do make the diagnosis correctly in the other 80 percent, they treat gestational diabetes with caloric restriction, insulin and sometimes drugs. This approach will always be flawed. We must treat the underlying problem, insulin resistance.

You'll remember in Chapter 5, we talked about a glucose/insulin (G/I) ratio that gives us a definitive diagnosis of insulin resistance and a more accurate picture of type 2 diabetes, and gestational diabetes as well. Impaired blood glucose tolerance because of insulin resistance is impaired glucose tolerance, whether you're pregnant or not.

The only good thing about gestational diabetes is that it usually goes into remission after the baby is born, although the risk of its return in later years is over 70 percent, because the underlying problem has not been treated. This underlying problem, insulin resistance, contributes to difficulty with weight loss and often continued weight gain after pregnancy. If the doctor would merely perform an insulin level test with every blood glucose test, elevated insulin levels and insulin resistance can be accurately diagnosed, treated and/or prevented in nearly every case. In my experience, a normal G/I ratio is over 20, 7–19 is reduced insulin sensitivity or increased resistance, and less than 7 is at least significant resistance, if not type 2 diabetes. The challenged test, getting blood tests simultaneously for glucose and insulin levels before and after a glucose load is most reliable, but an abnormal unchallenged test is highly significant in every case, and is more convenient and less costly.

Instead of these simple blood tests, conventional doctors merely rely on a blood glucose reading alone, which is often inaccurate in diagnosing the problem of significant insulin resistance. Then the physicians order a grueling three-hour glucose tolerance test in pregnancy (this is a two-hour test in nonpregnant women), again leaving out the all-essential information, you guessed it: the G/I ratio.

It is important to remember that in the practice of medicine, in most cases any abnormal test is more significant than a normal one. If the blood glucose level is above normal or the G/I ratio is below normal, this is significant in every case and implies significant insulin resistance. When diagnosing insulin resistance, ask your doctor to perform an insulin level test with every glucose level every time it is tested and calculate the G/I ratio every time a glucose level is taken. Once this level is known, it can be repeated less often just to insure improvement is being achieved. If this is not done, you risk missing the opportunity to learn if you have insulin resistance before it can hurt you.

Medical science tells us several things about what happens to a woman after multiple pregnancies:

- If a woman has repeated pregnancies that are less than 2 years apart, her risk of miscarriage and her baby's risk of birth defects increases.

- With each pregnancy, the risk of miscarriage and birth defects increases.

- As a woman ages, her risk of birth defects and miscarriages increases.

- If she has a previous pregnancy affected by a birth defect, her risk of having another is increased.

- If a woman has had more than three miscarriages, her rate of subsequent miscarriage goes up significantly.

- If her TSH (thyroid stimulating hormone) level is 2.5 or above, there is a 15 percent increased risk of miscarriage. This risk increases another 15 percent for every 1 point above that number. Remember, there is already a 15 percent risk of miscarriage in all pregnancies, so a "normal range" 3.5 TSH result would represent a 45 percent overall increased risk of miscarriage. Worst of all, her doctor might not even realize she has a thyroid problem and the increased risk to her baby. This is why there are so many articles now published regarding the adverse pregnancy effects of "borderline hypothyroidism." It is not "borderline"; it is the real thing. It's just not accurately diagnosed or treated. One would expect that since the symptoms are the same for all types of hypothyroidism, the consequences may also be the same.

- We know that babies' IQs are lower when the mothers' TSH levels are high. Unfortunately, we have no normal values for basal body temperatures in pregnancy; therefore, I try to be sure the TSH level is maintained at the lowest possible normal level (0.4 to 1.0).

- In addition, two large studies have also shown iodine supplementation can increase the child's IQ by over 10 points. In 1995 over 50 percent of all pregnant women in 18 states were found to be iodine deficient. This problem is probably much worse today with decreasing salt use and may be further compounded by the bromine issue, which may have further implications with regards to autism incidence. (We will discuss this further in Chapter 8.)

All of the above problems associated with multiple pregnancies are related to increasing nutritional deficiencies and accelerated mineral depletion with inadequate replacement and mineral imbalance.

Miscarriages are also related to mineral deficiencies. Also, it has been shown that over 70 percent of all miscarriages are related to chromosomal abnormality, which is nearly always associated with birth defects, as well as mental retardation. Almost all other serious birth defects, which cause infant death, are sporadic, not chromosomal. More than 50 percent of infant deaths in the United States are caused by one of these two factors. Imagine the impact if we merely treated the human animal as well as our farm animals are treated by providing all the missing and deficient minerals, not just calcium and the assorted other imbalanced chelated minerals as are found in the typical prenatal "vitamins"! This is an unnecessary tragedy obviously related to nutritional ignorance on the part of most, if not all, of our doctors.

What is the common denominator in all these circumstances? The common denominator in these sad scenarios is that the mother's deficient mineral storehouse has been consistently further depleted by her babies and she has not taken the time or the necessary minerals to regain or replace what she has lost. These mineral deficiencies and imbalances get worse with age and are rapidly depleted in pregnancy for all the reasons we have previously discussed: the lack of ionic minerals in our diet.

Imagine a woman who has had five children who potentially would have had her mineral storehouse depleted by over 50 percent! If she's like most women, she would not have started with optimal mineral levels and balance. It's hard to imagine how she could be walking around, much less caring for five kids and doing all the things that modern moms do. Life alone would make her tired, but when you consider the mineral depletion the pregnancies have caused and the increased thyroid resistance problem, it's no wonder so many women have problems with depression, weight, energy, migraines and hormones that increase in intensity after pregnancy.

It's also amazing how forgiving and adaptable the human body is. It never ceases to amaze me when I see someone who, on paper, looks like he/she should be at death's door, and he/she is actually coping rather well. Most of the things that cause our health to deteriorate happen slowly over time. Unfortunately, it is much harder to regain health than to keep it. Our health is our most valuable asset, our most precious resource. Never take your health for granted. The absence of a crisis does not mean you are healthy. Keep working at improving it daily. It is better to start now than wait for a health crisis or problem to develop. You don't have to be perfect, just be working at achieving better health every day. Knowing the information in this book can make a huge difference.

Teresa's Story

I think of Teresa as the candle lady because she always brought a small gift when she came to my office, for my staff or me. Often she gave us little candles, a thoughtful gesture we don't often see.

Teresa had great difficulty getting pregnant. She had suffered two early miscarriages and, at 38, she was afraid her biological clock was running down. Her HTMA showed a variety of mineral deficiencies and imbalances, and I thought her infertility might be related to her mineral status, so I started her on ionic minerals.

We all rejoiced when, four months later, we confirmed Teresa was pregnant.

Her pregnancy was routine until we got to the 22nd week, about five and one half months, when she began to gain weight rapidly. She had already eliminated dairy products from her diet, so I was concerned she might be showing signs of developing gestational diabetes. I ordered a glucose/insulin screen that wouldn't normally have taken place until six weeks further into her pregnancy.

The results came back as I had suspected: her glucose/insulin ratio was very low. A glucose tolerance test with insulin levels at every increment confirmed the diagnosis: Teresa had gestational diabetes. Needless to say, she was very worried since she had such difficulty conceiving, and she had successfully carried her baby through the first trimester when the risk of miscarriage is highest.

"What can I do, Dr. Thompson?" she pleaded with me as she dabbed at her eyes with a tissue.

I placed her on gradually increasing levels of ChromeMate, a patented nicotinic acid-bound form of chromium, with every meal. She also started on 100 percent whole-food vitamins and large amounts of trace minerals. She was testing her fasting blood sugars every morning and two hours after one of her largest meals of the day until her glucose readings were within the normal ranges.

It took about three weeks for Teresa to get her ChromeMate intake to the place where her sugars were normal. From there, it was smooth sailing. Her weight gain was within the expected amounts and she went on to deliver an 11-pound baby boy with completely normal blood sugars after birth. Teresa's sugars also remained normal even after the stress of the delivery.

As an interesting (and sad) aside, several of my fellow doctors and some of the nurses noticed that Teresa's and her baby's blood sugars were perfectly normal after delivery, but none of them asked me how this could be in a mother diagnosed with gestational diabetes, nor did they ask what I had done to address the problem. I volunteered the information, explaining the reason for the wonderful outcome for Teresa and her baby, but they just shrugged and dismissed it as an "unexplained" improvement.

The patient went on to lose her pregnancy weight and then some. Baby and Mom are beautifully healthy today and share their story often, but their success usually falls on deaf ears. Maybe the health concerns of pregnant women blind them to possibilities of better health, and they invariably tell Teresa they'll just follow their doctors' order. It's their loss and that of their precious babies.

These conditions are reversible. Time and time again, I've seen how quickly a woman can regain her mineral stores, her energy, her optimal weight and recover from blood sugar imbalances experienced during pregnancy with a simple regimen of the right minerals, supplements and eating habits based on HTMA results and knowing for sure.

Calcium problems

There are two more common complications of pregnancy that we haven't mentioned yet.

The first is pregnancy-induced hypertension or high blood pressure. In Chapter 4, we explained how the Calcium Cascade can lead to sodium/potassium membrane electrical potential failure (S/PMEP) and accelerate the process by which most patients experience high blood pressure, vascular dysfunction and a shortfall of nitric oxide production, the biochemical substance that dilates blood vessels. As with many complications of pregnancy, it's best to prevent them rather than to treat them, so getting your minerals and amino acids in balance before a pregnancy is your best bet. However, experts estimate that half of the pregnancies in the U.S. aren't exactly planned. So it's best to be at optimal mineral and nutritional levels all the time.

Another relatively unfamiliar complication is calcification of the placenta. This is most certainly contributed to by an excess of intracellular calcium in the placenta, inherited from the mother. The placenta is a fascinating organ, programmed to be born, serve its purpose of protecting and nourishing the fetus, and die in about 9.5 months. Because of its fast-forward life span, the placenta is a good reflection of general body health. If the placenta starts to harden (just like a hardening artery), the pregnancy is in trouble. If we see a fully mature placenta two, three or even four weeks before term or more, very often the baby isn't getting the nutrients it needs, growth starts to slow and sometimes we even have to deliver the baby early.

A slight blood pressure *drop* is a common standard at about 20 weeks of pregnancy. If that blood pressure drop doesn't occur or if the blood pressure is above normal early in pregnancy, I immediately put the mother on ionic minerals and shark liver oil (high in healthy fats and alkyl glycerols). In every case, for more than 12 years now, the blood pressure problems have been stopped and these pregnancies have continued normally.

Avoiding calcium excess, getting essential fatty acids and whole-food vitamins, especially the whole C vitamin (not ascorbic acid!), are the best ways to prevent both pregnancy-induced hypertension and calcification of the placenta.

I am absolutely convinced that every woman who becomes pregnant should have an HTMA test (if she hasn't already had one) and she, like nearly everyone else in the country and in the world, needs balanced ionic trace mineral supplements, at least 7.5 grams per day in pregnancy. In my experience, this treatment pretty much eliminates most high blood pressure complications in pregnancy. Since I learned about whole-food supplements, trace minerals and shark liver oil in 1996, I have not had a premature delivery because of hypertension or preeclampsia, if the mother came to me throughout her pregnancy and complied with my supplement regimen.

By the way, shark liver oil, high in alkyl-glycerols, is one of my most recommended supplements for hypertension. It causes blood pressures to become normal in about 50 percent of the patients who take it. Other fish oils do not work, or they don't work as well.

Thinking it through

Let's think about this for a moment.

We now know that most American adults have only about 5 percent to 20 percent of the intracellular sodium reserves we need, due to calcium excess inside their cells and lack of adequate sodium intake.

This includes pregnant women.

So when a woman becomes pregnant, she has only 5 percent to 20 percent of the sodium she needs to drive her S/PMEP and bring minerals, glucose and essential amino acids into all her body's cells, except fat cells.

She then passes on this depleted mineral status to her baby. She gets more critically nutritionally deficient as the pregnancy progresses. Worse yet, this level of deficiency increases with each subsequent pregnancy.

Perhaps one of the first things that happens is that the baby gets gas and indigestion in the first month of life. Already, the poor little tyke is experiencing protein digestive failure. Maybe the pediatrician even prescribes proton pump inhibitors. You can see where this is going. The Calcium Cascade (Chapter 2) is already taking place in a tiny baby!

What lies ahead for this little one?

We know that kids have poor eating habits today. My heart aches when I see what people feed their kids these days: comfort foods, fast foods, milk and juice by the gallon, even bromine-containing soft drinks and bakery goods. Wow! No wonder these kids are sick more often.

Over time, these little ones grow, but not as well or as healthy as they should be. We hear of more and more life-impacting sports injuries in Little Leaguers and young athletes that indicate vitamin C deficiency, and increasing allergy problems that indicate immune system compromise and dysfunction. I know that in Anchorage, Alaska, the number of children carrying epi-pens to school because of life-threatening allergies has increased by over 500 percent in the last ten years, suggesting an epidemic of immune system dysfunction.

By the time a child is in elementary school, there is a 30 percent chance he/she is overweight and has at least one chronic health problem.

The failure of protein digestion and the sodium/potassium membrane electrical potential failure can occur at an astonishingly young age. We know this because we are seeing more and more cases of metabolic failure, like type 2 diabetes, in young children and teens. Type 2 diabetes was once called adult-onset diabetes, but that name has become inaccurate, since so many children and teenagers are being diagnosed with the disease. Obesity is the common factor among almost every single child with insulin resistance, type 2 diabetes. Even before they become obese, almost all of these children have type 2 hypothyroidism.

You don't have to reread the earlier sections of this book to understand how failure to digest protein, S/PMEP failure and metabolic dysfunction lead to these problems. This is a national catastrophe of untold proportions. Once a 50- or 60-year-old might be diagnosed with type 2 diabetes and expect that in 10 to 20 years to experience the terrible diseases that accompany diabetes like heart disease, kidney failure, neuropathy, vision problems that lead to blindness, circulatory problems that cause poor wound healing and amputations. Today we face a much more grim reality.

Now think of a 15-year-old diagnosed with type 2 diabetes and with high cholesterol at 21. Fifteen years later, he is only 36 and already suffering from hypertension, morbid obesity and high cholesterol. Think of a 15-year-old-girl with the same problem and as soon as she has a baby, her mineral status is even further compromised. As teenagers, both of these hypothetical kids suffer from type 2 hypothyroidism and, by the age of 40, they are diabetic, hypertensive and in need of kidney transplant, heart bypass or gastric bypass surgery. Their life expectancies are dramatically shortened and the quality of what life they have left is poor. This is one of the reasons why experts say that, for the first time in modern history, our children's life expectancies may be shorter than our own.

Frightening, isn't it?

I actually find it exasperating, because all of this could quite simply be prevented and treated by increasing and balancing minerals, adding whole-food supplements and by making specific HTMA directed dietary changes. These are the basics. Without them, not much else matters.

Birth defects are often preventable

What would you say if I told you that I have a formula that could eliminate more than 50 percent of deaths of newborns, 98 percent of all birth defects and over 70 percent of miscarriage? Sounds crazy, but it makes total sense based on our farm animal data. This statement is based on the same basic biochemistry that any pre-med student must understand to proceed to medical school.

Half of the children born with major birth defects in the U.S. will die within the first six months of life. Statistically, those children with severe birth defects probably have little chance for survival, as sad as it may seem.

Some major birth defects are associated with carried genetic traits, but the majority have no predictive factors. Many other birth defects are caused by spontaneous chromosome abnormalities, like Down's syndrome. These two types of birth defect-related problems are the most likely preventable through aggressive balanced ionic trace mineral supplementation and balancing and by correcting vitamin C deficiency with whole versions of the nutrient.

This is where animal husbandry on the farm has made the greatest strides. Farmers have achieved a 70 percent reduction in miscarriage and a 98 percent reduction in birth defects with sea salt mineral supplementation in animals. I see no reason why this could not easily translate to the human experience. After 13 years of looking at HTMA results, I am willing to make any bet you like that this is true for humans as well. If we eliminate mineral deficiencies and imbalances before conception, 98 percent of these birth defects could be prevented. This would mean that we could reduce infant deaths by more than 50 percent in as little as one year through correct mineral and whole-food vitamin C supplementation and diet changes based on HTMA results. That means we could save 60,000 babies in the U.S. alone every year.

The other half of the children born with major birth defects typically have significant chromosome abnormalities and their associated birth defects. Somehow, these pregnancies escape miscarriage and the children go on to be born. It remains unclear as to whether mineral replacement could reduce or eliminate these birth tragedies.

There is no intervention in healthcare history that could have a greater impact on life and death. The death of a newborn has an impact that goes on for generations. The pain and suffering lasts a lifetime. The "fix" is embarrassingly cheap. We must give our children the healthiest possible start in life. This simple fix would also have a major impact on health care expenditures in the U.S. and throughout the world.

If we are smart enough to give our farm animals sea salt to prevent birth defects, why aren't we smart enough to do it for ourselves?

Several years ago, it was recognized that folic acid deficiency was a major factor in a birth defect called neural tube. The neural tube is a structure present in embryos that eventually develops into the central nervous system. Defects in the neural tube are developed in early pregnancy and can result in a variety of deformities in spine and brain development in children. What followed was a folic acid frenzy. It became a necessity in prenatal vitamins and the government mandated the addition of folic acid to common foods (primarily flours and cereals).

That is all supposed to be well and good. The Centers for Disease Control and Prevention (CDC) says that since 1996, when the Food and Drug Administration mandated the folic acid fortification program, the number of neural tube defects has declined by about 25 percent.

That's excellent, but it's only a tiny part of the whole picture. Neural tube defect is only one type of birth defect. Only about 2,500 babies are born in the U.S. each year with neural tube defects. About half of those are still linked to folic acid deficiency in mothers.

That is about 1 percent of the babies born with birth defects every year (about 4,000 babies per year). The March of Dimes estimates there are over 120,000 babies born with major birth defects in the U.S. each year, nearly 3 percent of all babies born or 3 percent of the 3,999,386 babies born in 2010. Birth defects are the leading cause of infant mortality in the U.S., accounting for over 20 percent of infant deaths according to the CDC.

The cause of over 70 percent of those birth defects is "unknown" to medical science. But I would suggest mineral deficiency and imbalance is a significant factor and probably includes the vitamin C molecule deficiency.

Telomeres for DNA replication also require adequate levels of selenium. The vitamin C molecule (not ascorbic acid) regenerates the biologic activity of selenium and selenium-rich proteins. Thyroid hormone production requires selenium, L-tyrosine, and whole-food vitamin C and copper. The body cannot utilize copper, metabolize cholesterol, make hemoglobin and a host of other biochemical essentials without whole-food vitamin C. Almost everything the human body does biochemically depends on these basic factors, pure water, minerals and whole-food vitamin C

I have no problem with the folic acid fortification program, but I think it doesn't go far enough. As with folic acid supplementation, this would be more effective if the supplementation began before the woman became pregnant, maybe even in the teenage years, since nearly 70 percent of mineral stores for life are determined during adolescence, and the majority of birth defects occur in the first month of pregnancy, often before a woman is even aware she is pregnant. Obviously, there are other factors to consider like environmental toxins and chemicals, but since minerals are a nutritional necessity for strong bones and good health, ongoing supplementation simply makes common sense.

Menopause

What we have covered in this chapter and the previous chapters applies very well to menopause. It is estimated that as many as 40 percent of perimenopausal (nearly menopausal) women have low thyroid function that adds to their symptoms when their hormones begin to fluctuate and full menopause approaches. I believe this statistic is way too conservative. More realistically, it is near 90 percent or more. Hypothyroidism is especially likely, nearly 95 percent, if the woman is more than 20 percent above her ideal body weight.

If you think back to the symptoms of types 1 through 5 hypothyroidism, with its fatigue, irritability, insomnia, weight gain, mood and energy swings and more, these sound remarkably like the symptoms of menopause. The symptoms of hormone deficiency often overlap or are similar in many cases for our endocrine hormones.

In addition, the major female hormones estrogen and progesterone lose their effectiveness when there is a zinc/copper imbalance, which frequently occurs with calcium excess and mineral imbalances or deficiencies. This is a problem with many of the "multidrug vitamins" where zinc and copper ratios are often improperly formulated, thus contributing to further hormone dysfunction. In fact, hormones also need minerals, especially iodine, in order to do their work. So when minerals are missing, displaced or out of balance, the hormones will be out of whack. Bromine also interferes with the iodine needed for all hormone functions. Add that to the hormonal fluctuations that begin as a woman nears the end of her child-

Bromine Is Not Your Friend!
(Skip this part if chemistry scares you)

I must briefly discuss the bromine issue here again because it is of such critical importance. This is a mineral, similar to iodine in its biologic properties, both halides on the periodic table of the elements. Unfortunately, bromine, a smaller atom with more electrons, has a significantly higher affinity for iodine binding sites in every cell in our bodies, in every biochemical reaction requiring iodine, and on every hormone molecule in the body, much more so than iodine. Therefore, it stands to reason that bromine will disrupt all iodine functions in the human body. There is simply no evidence that bromine is safe for use in humans.

Chlorine and fluorine also have some iodine interference effects in human physiology, but these are probably more temporary or less pronounced since these are smaller atoms than iodine with fewer electrons to grab onto substances in the body that already should have iodine atoms in their biochemical place. Therefore, they would not be as likely to displace the all important iodine atom from its all important biochemical or hormonal processes.

As it turns out, not only are thyroid hormones iodized, but so are ovarian hormones, pancreatic hormones and many other endocrine and secretory tissues and glands in the body that are all dependent on iodine for their biochemical functions. Therefore, bromine would be most likely to affect the endocrine organs and endocrine responsive tissues most severely. The ovary has the second highest concentration of iodine of any tissue in the human body. The breast tissue also uses significant amounts of iodine and is filled with endocrine responsive tissues.

Also and very importantly, every cell in our body uses iodine as part of the natural cell death process called "apoptosis." If iodine is replaced with bromine in these cellular equations, hormone dysfunction occurs and cell function is disrupted, cystic changes occur, apoptosis is reduced or inhibited, cells will not die and they are now called cancer cells. These cells go on to reproduce with unchecked growth and no normal apoptosis, a process due to lack of iodine or a block of iodine function by bromine. The evidence for this is compelling. Please refer to Dr. David Brownstein's books, *Iodine, Why You Need It, Why You Can't Live Without It*, and *Salt Your Way to Health*.

Unfortunately today and since 1980, bromine has been added to nearly all flour products instead of iodine, except King Arthur Flour, which specifically states "not brominated" on every label it sells. Bromine as methy bromide is also sprayed on our fruits, berries (especially strawberries, raspberries and blueberries), and some vegetables to prevent mold growth and extend shelf life.

Bromine is a mineral, so it's being sprayed on or put in our canned or jarred food and fruits and vegetables. Its use as a gas pesticide does not interfere with the "organic" label representation, which is basically only denoting the lack of organophosphates (pesticides, herbicides and organic fungicides). Unless the label of any jar, bottle, flour-containing product or produce specifically states, "not brominated," we have to assume bromine is in there.

Bromine is basically added to these canned foods and bottled drinks (soft drinks) to extend their shelf life. It is added to flour to keep it from clumping. Once again, since it is a mineral, it does not have to be listed on the label.

It is added to spas and swimming pools instead of the more easily evaporating chlorine.

It is hard to believe that this problem has gone largely unrecognized in the U.S. Australia banned the use of bromine in flour products in 2008. Unfortunately, they still allow it to be sprayed on their strawberries and who knows what else (as do all other agricultural countries). At least in Australia, they are beginning to recognize the problem and make this change. We seem incapable of making these necessary changes in the U.S. It seems we cannot get past protecting the status quo. I pray it is not just about big business and profits. Disease is unfortunately big business!

The effects of the hormonal and tissue biochemical disruption caused by the bromine mineral's interference with iodine are enormous. They include associations with nearly all fibrocystic breast disease, all cyclic and hormonal-related breast tenderness, breast cysts, dense breast tissue and many forms of breast cancer, all ovarian cysts. Most likely PMS, endometriosis and ovarian cancer may also all be attributed to or caused by bromine.

Bromine's ability to disrupt iodine function is also strongly implicated in thyroid dysfunction, autoimmune thyroiditis and thyroid cancer, as well as prostate cancer and maybe even pancreatic cancer. Incidentally, these are all hormone-producing endocrine glands or secretion-producing glands and hormone-responsive tissues, which are dependent on iodine to function normally. Epidemiologic data suggests that merely supplementing with iodine, at the level the Japanese consume daily or around 12.5 milligrams, reduces the incidence of breast cancer and prostate cancer by over 40 percent. That is a huge number! Iodine supplementation therefore becomes critical to long-term health as does avoiding bromine.

You can measure your iodine and bromine levels with an iodine challenge test, which I highly recommend. The bromine can then be eliminated from the body over time by taking large amounts of iodine daily until the bromine is reduced to its naturally occurring levels. Bromine has a half-life in the human body of 12 days. However, when sodium is deficient, this half-life is extended to over 96 days, an 800 percent increase, based on laboratory animal experiments. There are some reports of cancers simply disappearing with high doses of iodine alone.

We must start addressing this bromine issue right away. We simply cannot go on tolerating the high incidences of these cancers we now see in our loved ones. Bromine should be outlawed from our food, our drinks, our flour, our jars, cans, bottles and spas. Too many people are dying of prostate and breast cancer. This matter is of huge importance.

bearing years and her hormones start to spike and bottom out in unpredictable ways, and you get the picture.

To make matters worse, many menopausal women begin to take more and more calcium supplements because of the widely espoused fear of osteoporosis. We know that by taking calcium supplements, they are causing their mineral status to become more unbalanced and this accelerates the Calcium Cascade.

Bioidentical hormones

Finally, there are political and pharmaceutical forces afoot that are trying to take away a woman's right to use the only safe form of hormone replacement therapy, bioidentical hormones. These are the exact same hormones that replace the hormones already naturally occurring in women's bodies before menopause. They are exactly and purely bioidentical and given in the correct doses and balance.

There is no excuse for the FDA cowering to drug companies trying to stop the compounding of these bioidentical hormones. They are generic, not patentable, available only by prescription, FDA approved and they have been in use for more than 50 years. Physicians do however need to be educated about how to use these compounds correctly. Many have never even heard of them or seem to lack awareness of what bioidentical actually means.

Furthermore, there is quite simply no justification for the obvious discrimination against women with regard to hormone replacement, i.e., these medications are not covered by insurance companies or Medicare. This is a tragedy. These insurance companies are typically paying for testosterone replacement in men, and exorbitantly so, over 10 times the cost of this generic hormone that should cost pennies (nearly $300.00 per month for FDA-approved topical testosterone). Compounded generic hormones, in precise dosages based on hormone testing, cost my patients about $300 per year.

I disclosed my success with transmucosal bioidentical hormone replacement therapy (TMHRT, the state of the art) to the leadership of the American College of OB/GYN meeting in 2011 and asked that the college consider studying my work. Sadly, they were not interested. The American Academy of Anti-Aging Medicine has shown some interest.

Unfortunately, there is very little understanding in the field of women's health as to how to replace these hormones safely and effectively. So many women and even doctors are so confused about what it means to get bioidentical hormones that they remain stuck in their ignorance. They continue to compare apples to oranges thinking that the research on the drugs that "act like hormones," which are chemical patentable substances, will have the same effects as the actual bioidentical hormones that naturally exist in the human. Misinformation is rampant and leadership is lacking.

Except in women's health, there are quite simply no other examples in the entire field of medicine where a specific hormone would be replaced with something other than the exact hormone needed. We would not and should not even consider giving some chemical that "acts like" or has some properties of or "effects like" those of a hormone that we found the need to replace in the human. At least, we wouldn't consider it if we were thinking. There is simply no justification for these drugs that are not human hormones that we ob-gyn physicians have given to our patients innocently, but mistakenly, for over 50 years. We were misled and not thinking. We should have known better.

Now we need to admit our mistake and do it right more than ever. We are simply letting our society suffer from the consequences of these deficiencies without a conscience. Hormone replacement must be done with bioidentical and correctly formulated physiologic doses and balances (not therapeutic doses like the suppressive dose of birth control pills) of the exact same hormones that we would naturally have in our bodies when healthy.

Every single disease process of aging, including cancer, heart disease and dementia to name a few, without exception has been shown to be reduced with this approach. There is simply no remaining controversy, just ignorance.

I'm not much of an activist, but the opposition of the drug companies to bioidentical compounding is just plain outrageous. This greedy, most blatant effort by drug companies to squelch the bioidentical hormone "competition" should be condemned. If all of us, especially women, don't fight back, we'll all lose. You can contact your elected officials through the FANS (Freedom of Access to Natural Solutions) website at: www.project fans.org/law-legislation.cfm.

Never, ever take synthetic or equine-based "hormones." These are chemical substances that act like "hormones" isolated from the urine of pregnant mares, and they contain estrogen compounds that have never ever been found naturally in women's bodies. Most notably, these are Premarin (PREgnantMAResʼ urINe) and Prempro, which contains Premarin and a synthetic "progesterone" (which is actually a testosterone derivative). Beware of all progestins: They are typically testosterone derivatives, and not anything like the naturally occurring hormone progesterone. These drugs act like hormones and have been proven in large studies not only to increase the risk of breast cancer and blood clotting, but they dramatically increase the risk of heart attack, stroke and Alzheimer's disease. Don't do it! Remember, there is no acceptable comparison of these chemicals to bioidentical hormones that naturally exist, safely in women's bodies.

Now here's the zinger: Guess who filed the complaint that attempted to end the era of compounding pharmacies and bioidentical hormone replacement? Wyeth Pharmaceuticals, the manufacturer of Premarin and Prempro. That's the same company whose sales suddenly plummeted into the toilet after research proved their products were downright dangerous to women. So far they have lost $1 billion or more in sales. And they are still trying to justify the use of their dangerous drug!

These were products that had been in use for over 50 years, and virtually every doctor had been brainwashed into believing these horse-estrogens would *protect* women from osteoporosis, heart disease and strokes. The Premarin Lie has probably killed hundreds of thousands of women over the past 60 years. And now Wyeth wants to kill the competition, the place where many women have turned for safe hormone replacement. It's an outrage!

Interestingly, Wyeth, with the consent of the FDA, is doing this in the name of "safety and protecting the public." And they are getting away with it, so far. This company should be ashamed and so should the politicians and FDA bureaucrats who have listened to their lobbying efforts. In my opinion, Wyeth should be banned from selling products related to women's health forever and should be fined billions of dollars to be held in trust specifically for the treatment and care of those suffering from having received their drugs. They care only about money. They have misled enough doctors and patients and caused enough death and heartache already! Worse yet, they have yet to be held accountable.

Sadly, this is a common state of affairs in the pharmaceutical industry in general. Disease is big business and Big Pharma has every incentive to keep us sick.

POINTS TO REMEMBER

✔ Pregnant women lose approximately 10 percent of their total body mineral supply to their babies. That means each pregnant woman loses around four pounds of minerals to her baby with each pregnancy.

✔ Too many pregnancies too close together can severely compromise the mother's health and increase the risk of birth defects, which appear to be related at least in part to excessive mineral loss.

✔ Babies are programmed to take the minerals they need, even if the mother can't afford to lose them, because of their own deficiencies and imbalances.

✔ Babies are born with a near exact fingerprint of their mother's mineral status.

✔ Imbalanced minerals on the part of the mother are passed on to the baby, resulting in mineral imbalances and deficiencies from birth.

✔ Infants and young children also suffer the effects of calcium excess and mineral imbalances and deficiencies. These problems increase throughout a lifetime, due to the lack of ionic minerals in the diet, continued mineral losses, calcium excess in the diet and repeated family eating habits.

✔ Birth defects can be reduced by nearly 98 percent, if not nearly completely eliminated, miscarriage can be reduced by over 70 percent and infant death rates can be reduced by over 50 percent with adequate ionic trace mineral supplementation.

✔ Many of the problems women experience with menopause are attributable to calcium excess with type 2 hypothyroidism, impaired protein digestion with intracellular amino acid deficiencies and sodium/potassium membrane electrical potential failure with disruption of cellular function. Mineral balancing and appropriate nutritional corrections based on HTMA results and balanced physiologic doses of bioidentical hormones will keep hypothyroidism, weight gain, depression, irritability, hormone deficiency symptoms and insomnia at bay and greatly improve the quality of life of all men and women.

✔ There is overwhelming biological evidence that bioidentical hormone replacement is not only natural and safe, but it improves the quality of life and reduces not only breast cancer incidence, but it also reduces heart disease, stroke, dementia, osteoporosis, high cholesterol and almost every known chronic illness associated with aging.

✔ Balanced physiologic transmucosal bioidentical hormone replacement should replace every other mistaken form of hormone replacement therapy. The accuracy and reliability of this approach is so significant that it will change hormone replacement in medicine forever as knowledge of its use in anti-aging medicine spreads.

✔ Due to bromine toxicity across our entire population, iodine supplementation is a must to protect the brains of developing babies and to help reduce at least five different types of cancer (breast, prostate, ovarian, thyroid and pancreatic) as much as 40 percent or more. Please lobby our government to get bromine out of our food.

CHAPTER 7

The Vitamin Lie

W E ALL KNOW WE NEED VITAMINS in order to survive. Without minerals, none of these vitamins, sometimes called coenzymes, can be used by the human body, since minerals are part of the electrical transport system that brings the vitamins into the cells where they are needed.

Minerals are also needed to donate the electrons for all biochemical reactions that vitamins help to take place. Vitamins simply do not work without minerals. Furthermore, vitamins cannot be formed without minerals and trace minerals.

So, not only do we all need minerals in the proper balance, we also need vitamins. Imbalances in both vitamins and minerals can cause disease, pure and simple. Getting too much of a single vitamin or specific mineral can be just as dangerous as getting too little. Sometimes it's hard to know exactly what we need.

Here's the shocking crux of The Vitamin Lie: Almost all vitamins sold on the market today are not vitamins. They are drugs. Yes, drugs! How could this be?

Let's start with a couple of simple definitions:

What is a vitamin? A vitamin is a naturally occurring essential nutrient that either the body manufactures or the body derives from food or other sources (such as sunlight and HDL cholesterol in the case of vitamin D hormone). Vitamins are complex molecules, combinations of enzymes, amino acids and various trace minerals. They are food and should have no toxicity or adverse effects at any level, contrary to common belief.

What is a drug? It's a chemical compound that does not normally occur in the human body. Drugs are chemical substances synthesized by laboratories. Drugs may have some basis in naturally occurring nutrients, but they have been synthetically or chemically altered, broken into pieces, and are not biochemically identical to the naturally occurring complex vitamin molecules or hormones that naturally exist in our bodies.

Vitamin C in drug form can be fatal

Vitamin C is a great example. Vitamin C is absolutely essential to human survival. We'll go into this in much greater detail in the coming pages, but *vitamin C is not ascorbic acid,* despite what most of us have been led to believe. Yes, ascorbic acid is one of many nutrients in the vitamin C molecule. I sometimes refer to it as being like the address on an envelope. It gets it there, but doesn't do anything. We have to open the envelope to see what's inside. The *whole C molecule* is what we really need and, as you'll see in the coming pages, ascorbic acid alone actually depletes vitamin C from the body and can even be quite dangerous when given to people who are severely vitamin C-deficient.

Vitamin C complex molecules also contain P, K and J factors, the tyrosinase enzyme, at least 14 known bioflavonoids, various ascorbagens, five copper ions, iron, manganese, zinc, selenium, phosphorus, magnesium and yes, ascorbic acid. Nutrient vitamins like vitamin C are extremely complex molecules and there are probably dozens, if not hundreds, of other nutrients present in this molecule that we have not yet discovered.

The body is completely dependent on the whole vitamin C molecule. We cannot make it ourselves, so we must get it from our food in order for us to survive. There is no evidence that fragments of that molecule have any of the same effects as the whole C molecules.

It is pretty simple: Biochemically, ascorbic acid is nothing like vitamin C. It is a pro-oxidant, not an antioxidant, meaning it causes oxidation in the body. Think of rust on a car's bumper. That's oxidation. It's not good when it happens to your cells. Ascorbic acid is much more like an antibiotic than a vitamin. It works by inducing the production of hydrogen peroxide (H_2O_2) or by increasing ROS (reactive oxygen substances) inside the body's cells. This gives ascorbic acid very specific antiviral, antibacterial, and possibly anticancer properties, like drugs. There is no longer any confusion except in the name: Ascorbic acid is a drug. There might be times when its short-term use is appropriate, but ascorbic acid is *not* vitamin C. It actually depletes C. Referring to "vitamin C" as ascorbic acid has confused, para-lyzed, distorted, and flawed all research regarding the actual vitamin C mol-ecule. I refer to this as The Vitamin C Lie.

Ascorbic acid has completely different effects than the whole C molecule. Ascorbic acid (a smaller lighter molecule) competes for the bind-ing sites for vitamin C on our cells and causes the excretion of the real C molecule in the urine. Ascorbic acid quickly depletes our body's stores of this life-giving all-important vitamin C molecule. I am not sure if there is a single worthwhile benefit to ascorbic acid when one considers the impact of the ascorbic acid molecule on the total body depletion of the real vita-min C molecule from our bodies. Please hear me. If you have been getting IV "vitamin C" or taking large doses of ascorbic acid, quit right away and begin taking the real C molecule. Your life and health depend on making this change. If you do not, you will continue to suffer from vitamin C defi-ciency problems.

But here's the economic reality: Almost all "vitamin C" on the market today is ascorbic acid or variations thereof. It says so right on the label in the parentheses, "vitamin C (as ascorbic acid)." Why? Ascorbic acid is incredibly cheap to synthesize and/or isolate in a lab, with very little or no natural plant material.

Vitamins cannot be patented, so drug and supplement companies have no interest in producing quality, whole-food products upon which they can expect to make little profit. They know we have bought into The Vitamin Lie and that most of us believe we must have "vitamin C" to prevent colds and a host of other maladies, so they know we'll buy it. What you don't know is that, at best, the ascorbic acid you bought at the drug store is in reality doing almost nothing good for you. It is actually depleting your total body vitamin C levels. Ascorbic acid (not C) makes the signs and symptoms of the real vitamin C deficiency worse. In the treatment of scurvy (called "the hemorrhagic disease" in the past from extreme and prolonged vitamin C deficiency), ascorbic acid will make the problem worse, if not fatal. This is called the "reverse effect."

Tiny pieces of a whole food

"Vitamin C" (as ascorbic acid) is only one of the multitudes of so-called "vitamins" and their derivatives and combination formulas on the market today that qualify as drugs. They are not natural, no matter what the label says. These are only tiny pieces of the whole-food that is the source of the vitamin you need. Vitamins are extremely complex molecules, most of them with more components than science has yet been able to detect.

For example, vitamin A is actually a family of three groups of biochemical compounds (retinoids, retinols and retinoic acids) and there are over 600 known forms of retinoids alone, with at least 19 of these found in the human body. Only one of these, the beta-carotene molecule, is the part that is present in most synthetic forms of "vitamin A." These nutrient components work synergistically. In simple terms, this means that the whole is greater than the sum of the parts: Each little component of a vitamin molecule enhances the function of the others.

It's another "aha!" moment when we realize how whole-foods are designed to contain *all* the nutrients our bodies need.

Think of it this way: If you take ascorbic acid or beta-carotene or another single component of a "vitamin," it's like taking calcium only when your body needs all 76 ionizing salt-form minerals for survival. Calcium is a necessary mineral for everyone, but to take calcium without all the other minerals or to take one mineral in excess, is inviting disaster, as you've learned in the earlier chapters of this book.

Along the same lines, to take part of a vitamin without taking the whole vitamin invites similar disaster. Any vitamin you take should be carefully collected from whole-foods that have been vineripened in minerally balanced soil and picked at their nutritional peak. In addition, they should be alcohol extracted and processed without heat, which is a notorious destroyer of these delicate life-sustaining nutrients.

How to find the right real vitamin

How do you know if your vitamins meet these requirements? That's the $64,000 question considering the artificial need that drug and supplement companies have created for products that aren't what they promise. Buyer beware! Your health is at stake.

Here are my suggestions:

- If the label doesn't tell you that your product is made from vine-ripened, organically produced, alcohol-extracted whole-foods, without heat, it probably is not of the quality you are seeking. It is a drug. You can request a certificate of analysis (COA) from the marketing company to confirm that the product they are marketing is the true bioidentical whole-food molecule in its intact form. Most reputable companies worth their "salt" (pun intended), will be able to produce a COA from an independent source that confirms that what they are selling you is the intact bioidentical whole-food vitamin molecule.

- Here's another great clue: If the label says vitamin C (as ascorbic acid) or vitamin A (as beta-carotene), don't waste your money. Those parentheses mean a substitution has been made; only one piece of the whole-food molecule is in your multi, even if it says organic, whole-food derived or natural. If it costs $10 at your drug store, it definitely is not whole-food or truly a vitamin. It will actually deplete your body of the real thing or interfere with its actual vitamin functions. These drug form "vitamins" may actually have other effects, different from the real molecule, and thereby may be harmful. Conversely, if it says 100 percent whole-food and costs $30 to $70 at your local health food store, or enlightened doctor's office, it still may not be what you need, but you're on the right track. Whole-food vitamins cost a bit more, but they are definitely worth it because you are worth it. To take anything else is to waste your money and possibly to jeopardize your health.

- Check out the resources section of this book and look at our website — www.calciumlie.com—for recommendations on quality products and for updates, blogs and expanded information.

- If you're in doubt and you have a product in mind, contact the company and ask about contents, growing conditions and processing.

Take your vitamins and minerals separately. Avoid "multivitamins" that have minerals added. These added minerals are usually undissolvable, poorly absorbed and they may be harmful to you. Based on your tissue mineral levels, if you already have an excess of any one or more of the minerals typically added to your "multivitamin," that "vitamin" would be contraindicated. Your mineral needs should be determined by your hair tissue mineral analysis (HTMA) results, which are essential for correct supplementation. Your mineral intake should be carefully balanced so the vitamins can get the minerals where they are needed and both can do their jobs.

Don't pay attention to the government's RDAs or recommended daily allowances or RDIs, recommended daily intakes for "vitamins." I don't think anyone really knows the basis for these government-recommended amounts of "nutrients," but at least one author has theorized that they came from the nutrient profile of the needs of a World War I soldier, later revised and translated to women's needs without any scientific basis! How absurd! Considering the relative nutrient status of some 90-plus years ago, and the comparatively primitive nature of the laboratory equipment of the time, it makes absolutely no sense to conclude such a determination could apply to today's humans.

Today, the Food and Nutrition Board of the National Academy of Sciences meets every five years and sets or readjusts the RDAs. I find it difficult to understand how these intelligent people can be so misled. RDAs should not be confused with the needs or requirements for a specific individual. The key is to consume 100 percent whole-food vitamins and balanced mineral supplements.

The value of food

Of course, you should eat foods that provide the greatest amounts of the nutrients you need, hopefully based on a reliable tissue mineral analysis. Vine-ripened, fresh, fresh frozen, naturally dried, fermented and raw foods grown in mineral-rich soils generally contain the perfect proportions and perfect balance of most of the nutrients we all need.

There are problems with this, as you might imagine. Few of us eat exactly as we should. Most of us eat what we like and do so repetitively. Most of us eat about 20 foods over and over when there are literally thousands available to us. We eat what we grew up liking and what our parents fed us. We buy what we like every time we go to the store, so we grow up and develop "hereditary" nutritional medical problems. These are not inherited family medical problems or tendencies, but family-based nutritional habits that translate into nutritional imbalances and deficiencies and mineral imbalance and deficiency diseases—what I call Familial Nutritional Diseases.

It is difficult to avoid junk foods, fast foods and processed foods that are downright harmful to our health. Even if you're getting the greatest foods possible, grown locally without pesticides or other harmful chemicals, vineripened and shipped a short distance to your table while the nutrients are still at peak value, you're still probably missing essential minerals and vitamins.

Having a well-balanced diet with adequate minerals is a nice thought, but it's not very realistic. We already know that our mineral-depleted soil makes it nearly impossible to get all of our essential nutrients through food, and the majority of our food is not vine ripened. That makes supplements a necessary part of our nutritional system in order to make up the shortfalls. This doesn't mean you can compensate for a cheeseburger and chocolate cake diet by taking a few vitamins and minerals. Good nutrition is still and always at the heart of good health.

After 13 years and nearly 2000 HTMA results, I am convinced that it is nearly impossible to truly "eat to be healthy" due to the lack of nutrients in our soil and in our food. Unfortunately, it is very easy to eat to become unhealthy. We must supplement and do so correctly based on HTMA results and basic whole-food nutritional needs. The absence of a health crisis today does not mean we are healthy. We have to keep working at being healthy every day. This eventually becomes a lifestyle choice.

Remember, little changes lead to bigger ones. Supplementing correctly once per day leads to a 33 percent improvement in our healthfulness, twice per day a 66 percent improvement and three times per day a 99 percent improvement in our health provided the correct supplements are taken. If one good nutritional change is made, it will usually lead to two, then four, then more. I call this *healthful congruence*. Soon, other positive life changes occur. We really can feel better than we ever expected. But don't put it off, start today.

So, OK, you've got your minerals balanced and now it's time to go on to discuss the best vitamins. Here are the ABCs, and beyond, of what's good—and what's not and why.

ABCs of vitamins

There are five different classes of vitamin compounds or vitamin complexes. It's important that you remember that vitamins are complex and they are never, ever made up of one single nutrient.

Here are the basics of the A, B, C, D, E, F, G, and K's of vitamins:

Vitamin A

Here's what vitamin A does:

- Maintains health of immune system;
- Regulates inflammation, tissue repair and wound healing;
- Formation of skin cells and mucous membranes throughout the respiratory, digestive, urinary and genital tracts;
- Formation of bones and soft tissues, including muscles, cartilage and ligaments;
- Assists in adrenal and thyroid gland function;
- Essential for good eyesight, night vision and corneal health;
- Formation of tooth enamel;
- Assists in maintaining a normal pregnancy and embryonic development;
- Assists in reproduction, fertility, lactation, sperm and egg formation;
- Supports nervous system;
- Protects liver.

Dietary sources of the fat-soluble vitamin A include meat and cheese, red, orange and yellow fruits and vegetables, and dark green, leafy vegetables. Fish oils, egg yolk and butter are excellent natural fatty sources of this fat-soluble vitamin.

Vitamin A is actually a complex family of nutrients that includes retinols, retinoic acid and retinoids. There are actually over 600 known different kinds of retinoids, generally referred to as provitamins; 19 different ones have been found in humans, among them a group called beta carotenoids.

Vitamin A is *not* beta-carotene, although that is what you'll see on most vitamin bottles: "vitamin A (as beta-carotene)." Beta-carotene is a drug and has, in fact, been shown to cause increased risk of birth defects. The medical establishment has largely removed beta-carotene from prenatal vitamins because of its direct link to birth defects. This should have been a clue that something was wrong. Unfortunately, physicians have bought into The Vitamin Lie for so long, they didn't recognize the warning sign or the difference either. This shocked me when I first learned it since I too had been giving my patients prenatal vitamins with beta-carotene in them without questioning the label.

Like most physicians, I assumed that prenatal "vitamins" were the best of all vitamin products made for the protection of two lives, not just one. After all, some higher "intelligence" had apparently decided what to put in there. Unfortunately, when I did my homework, I realized they were downright harmful. They are basically drugs not vitamins.

Too much beta-carotene as found in our so-called vitamins can also cause hair loss, cirrhosis of the liver, water retention, skin diseases and many more unpleasant problems. Yet, you could drink carrot juice all day long, to the point where your skin turns orange, and while you might look a little strange, you wouldn't have any physical problems and if you're pregnant, it would not cause birth defects in your developing child. That's because the carotenoid-rich carrot juice is a whole-food. The beta-carotene found in carrots is a provitamin or precursor of vitamin A and is stored up in the body (liver, fat and skin) and only converted to vitamin A as it is needed. Vitamin A in its whole-food form has no known toxicity. It is 100 percent whole-food and not a drug. This is one of the strongest examples we have in the difference between these chemically isolated compounds (drugs) and organic 100 percent whole-food vitamins.

B Complex Vitamins

Most of us know that vitamin B isn't just one vitamin, but most of us think there are just 12 B vitamins. You'd probably be surprised to know there are at least 56 vitamins in the B family. These water-soluble vitamins are most commonly known as B1 (thiamine), B2 (riboflavin), B3 (niacinamide), B5 (pantothenic acid), B6 (pyridoxine), B7 (biotin), B9 (folic acid) and B12 (cobalamin). These vitamins are frequently referred to as "B-complex," although most of the drugs sold as "vitamins" contain only the most common B drug form "vitamins" and not the whole B vitamin complex molecules. While all of the components of the B-complexes can be separated, they always occur together in nature and no single B vitamin is ever found alone in a food.

Here's what the B vitamins do:

- They have a vital function in cellular metabolism as coenzymes to speed up biochemical processes;

- They help form DNA, the genetic material from which all cells are created and reproduce;

- They are necessary for the health and normal function of the nervous system;

- They maintain healthy skin, heart, liver, eyes, hair, spleen, thymus, pancreas, kidneys, red blood cell production and muscles;

- They stimulate digestion, secretion of digestive enzymes and insulin

- They are essential for immune system function, resistance to infection and injury;

- They are a key part of endocrine gland system function (thyroid, adrenals, pituitary, ovaries and testes);

- Promote cell growth and division, including healthy red blood cells;

- They facilitate carbohydrate, protein and fat metabolism, and cellular energy production;

- As a complex, they work synergistically to reduce and prevent stress, depression and cardiovascular disease.

B vitamins are found in clams, salmon, halibut, trout, salmon, beef, dairy products, brown rice, eggs, raw seeds and nuts, peas, avocados, nutritional yeast, bananas, oranges, grapes, pears, barley, oats, yams, corn, rye, dried beans, peppers of all types, dark green leafy vegetables, potatoes, tomatoes, and one of the best sources of all, stabilized rice bran.

Strict vegetarians and gastric bypass patients need B12 supplements, since the essential factor, methyl-tetra-hydro-cyanocobalamin, is found only in animal products and gastric bypass patients are typically unable to absorb it.

Any kind of refining, cooking or processing damages the molecular structures of the B-complex vitamins, which is again why raw foods are the best sources of vitamins.

I prefer to use raw seeds and nuts (use raw nuts only if you are at your ideal body weight because of their high caloric values), which contain good amounts of the B-complex vitamins undamaged by a heating process. Sprouts are also a good source of B-complex vitamins.

Would you pay for a tune up for your car and change only one spark plug? If you have several kids, would you feed only one? Would you pay for cable TV if there were only one channel? Taking only one B vitamin is neither logical nor efficient. So avoid doing it unless there is a good reason. Get your B vitamins from whole-foods. There is such a close relationship between the various B vitamins that a shortfall or excess of any one of this complex will affect the functions of all the other B vitamins. Large doses of one of the synthetic "vitamins" can also create an imbalance and cause a relative deficiency of other members of the B complex.

The need for whole-foods is underscored by the story of World War II American troops held in Japanese prisoner-of-war camps who were being fed a diet of white rice only. They were getting beriberi, a severe thiamine deficiency disease that results in nerve and heart damage, lack of coordination, numbness, stumbling gait, degeneration of nerve tissue, loss of reflexes, memory loss, loss of muscle tone, nausea, emotional instability, confusion, depression and leg edema. The situation became so dire that the Red Cross was given permission to bring in vitamin B1 (thiamine) to help them. But the Red Cross B1 vitamin didn't work, precisely because they contained a drug form of the thiamine alone. In fact, the symptoms got worse. What did work? It was tiny handfuls of rice bran given to prisoners by their more compassionate guards. The POWs found that four men could share one tiny rice kernel and get enough of the B-complex vitamins from the powder between the kernels of rice and the husk covering the kernels that they needed to maintain their health, or at least enough to reverse the severe thiamine deficiency symptoms.

Interestingly, stabilized rice bran is now available worldwide. This substance, obtained from the powderlike substance found between the kernels of rice and the husk could easily be the most healthful supplement on earth. It is loaded with B1, B3 and B6 in the whole-food form as well as over 69 other nutrients and 2 grams of fiber per serving. It helps lower cholesterol (whole-food B3 and 2 grams of soluble fiber per serving), improves thyroid function (whole-food B1), improves adrenal function and helps the liver, the heart, the brain and nearly every other organ in the body at a minimal cost, around $5.00 per 18-ounce bag.

I think this example can be translated to many Westerners today who subsist on a diet of processed and nutritionally void foods with few nutrients, including B-complex. That gives us another explanation for the widespread depression, anxiety, fatigue, neurological disorders, neuropathy, intestinal disorders and adrenal insufficiency, to name a few of the problems, that we see on a regular basis in our society.

The above is a brief discussion of only one form of B-complex vitamin. There are more than 50 other B vitamins. It's important to understand that no natural vitamin exists as a single chemical entity. Separated from their whole-food complex molecules, the single-structure chemical "vitamin" has had numerous coenzyme factors removed that are essential for the actions of these vitamins in humans.

Vitamin C

I'm sure you've already gotten the message that quite clearly vitamin C is perhaps the most important vitamin nutrient available to us as humans, but only in its whole-food form. It is the one vitamin deficiency that, in a severe form, will eventually kill you. We've already gone into vitamin C as an example, but this important nutrient complex bears much further examination. Ascorbic acid, a component of vitamin C, serves as the molecule's antioxidant envelope, where it protects the other nutrients in the molecule from deterioration. Ascorbic acid is only as much a representative of vitamin C as the wrapper is part of your candy bar. It's holding in and protecting the "good stuff" inside.

Here's what the components of the vitamin-C complex molecule do:

- **Rutin** (also called the **"P" factor**) strengthens blood vessels and other collagen containing tissues, like cartilage;

- The **"K" factor** supports proper blood clotting, much like vitamin K; it also limits bruising and contributes to bone strength;

- The **"J" factor** supports the oxygen-carrying capacity of the blood to the benefit of all organs and tissues;

- **Tyrosinase** activates organic or ionic copper, allowing copper to function in stimulating metabolism, energy production, hemoglobin formation, thyroid hormone production and cholesterol metabolism;

- The five **copper** ions per molecule along with the enzyme tyrosinase are needed to help iron to be incorporated into the hemoglobin molecule for healthy red blood cells, correcting anemia and activating the cytochrome P-450 oxidase system with the help of tyrosinase to metabolize cholesterol;

- The numerous **bioflavonoids** have numerous enzyme and metabolic cofactor actions, many of which are still unknown;

- **Ascorbagens** have beneficial effects on some liver and intestinal enzymes;

- **Ascorbic acid** is the binding site and part of the capsule of the molecule and has some antibiotic-like activity;

- The entire complex intact molecule is the key to nearly all metabolic processes in the human body;

- It is involved in the formation of collagen, which forms connective tissues, gives them strength and is responsible for many cellular functions, including skin health and wound healing;

- Immune system function is dependent on vitamin C-complex;

- Hormone actions and synthesis are dependent on C-complex;

- It assists in amino acid metabolism and absorption;

- Regenerates the active form of vitamin E complex.

Vitamin C is found primarily in vine-ripened citrus fruits, berries, peppers, cantaloupe, broccoli, sweet potatoes, cauliflower, pineapple and mangos. Vitamin C is easily destroyed by heat, so it's best to eat these foods raw. All store-bought juices, whether fresh or frozen, have to be pasteurized by law. That means they are heated to 162° F for at least 30 seconds. This heat literally explodes the C molecule, completely destroying its nutritional value.

Vitamin C deficiency is sadly one of the most significant health problems we face in our society today after mineral deficiency, largely because we've fallen prey to a subset of The Vitamin Lie, The Ascorbic Acid Lie. Our belief that vitamin C is ascorbic acid has led to an overall lack of consciousness of some of the functions of the C-complex molecule, including its role in blood clotting, immune function, connective tissue strength and healing. So we pop a handful of ascorbic acid tablets at the first signs of a cold and think that will take care of the problem.

It was Linus Pauling, the brilliant Nobel Prize laureate, who woke us up to the value of the vitamin C molecule, but Pauling used whole vitamin C in his research, not ascorbic acid.

When you take ascorbic acid to ward off a cold, you are actually getting an antibiotic or druglike effect of the drug ascorbic acid, not vitamin C. You also deplete the whole-food molecule, the real vitamin C complex molecule, from your body, shunting it off along with all of its other beneficial parts into your urine, without leaving behind anything good.

Conventional doctors pooh-pooh the idea that vitamin C deficiency is widespread in today's society. They think they haven't seen a case of scurvy in over 200 years since the link between citrus fruits and the sailors' vitamin deficiency was established and the potato blight of the 1800s occurred.

So what are the symptoms of scurvy? Thin skin, frequent bruising, bleeding from old wounds or even scars, purple swollen gums, bleeding gums, pale skin, fatigue, thinning hair, premature graying, poor wound healing, weak tissues, elevated cholesterol, thin skin, muscle and joint aches and pains, connective tissue weakness, among others. Doctors see it every day; they just don't recognize it as symptomatic of vitamin C deficiency.

Have you ever seen an elderly person with thinning hair and thin skin that bruises and breaks and bleeds easily? Perhaps she is losing her teeth or he's getting frequent nosebleeds or has large (bruises) on the arms or legs. Of course, older people nearly always complain of fatigue and body aches and pain. We're all related to someone like that and maybe we've even suffered some of those symptoms ourselves. Patients often tell me, "I bruise easily." All of these problems are signs of vitamin C complex deficiency and all of them are easily and quickly corrected with whole-food C-complex.

You don't have to be elderly to experience C-complex deficiency. Vitamin C is crucial to the production of soft tissues, like cartilage and ligaments and tendons. We're seeing injuries to these tissues in many teenagers and people in their 20s and 30s. Joint replacement has become common in people in their 40s and 50s because of their weak and deteriorating soft tissues due to vitamin C deficiency. Back problems and herniated discs are the product of the same deficiencies and result in millions of surgeries and spine and back interventions. Elevated cholesterol and plaque in your arteries from connective tissue weakness is also a sign of chronic C deficiency, which is caused in part or contributed to by taking ascorbic acid that depletes C from the body, as well as not getting the real C vitamin in our food.

In addition to your whole-foods C-complex, you'll need to increase your intake of C-rich foods. I eat at least half an orange every single day, even though I know it came from Florida or California all the way to Alaska. Sorry, we just can't grow oranges in Alaska. The thick skin of oranges helps preserve the vitamin content and most oranges are tree-ripened before they are picked, since they won't ripen off the tree. I fortify my orange drink in the morning with fresh frozen rose hips I pick every year in Alaska, and fresh frozen raspberries also picked from my raspberry patch, along with rice bran and fiber added. It's so good!

You know I'm really passionate about the importance of real vitamin C. Here's a rundown of what happens when you are deficient in this vital nutrient.

1. **Elevated cholesterol:** Our bodies cannot metabolize cholesterol without the real C molecule, which is required for copper utilization. It is logical to conclude that all persons with elevated cholesterol are vitamin C deficient. Having elevated cholesterol is more likely a vitamin C molecule deficiency problem, not a statin drug deficiency problem.

2. **Chronic anemia:** Our bodies cannot make hemoglobin without the C molecule and the mineral copper, which cannot be utilized in the body without the real vitamin C. It is pretty amazing how fast a lifelong anemia corrects with the real C molecule being given on a regular basis. Iron, although necessary, is much less important than the C molecule.

3. **Hemorrhage and easy bruising:** Blood cannot clot without the C molecule and, without C, tissues become fragile and vessels break easily. This is why scurvy was known as "hemorrhagic disease," from severe and prolonged vitamin C–molecule deficiency.

   This is the reason, in my opinion, for the increased maternal death from hemorrhage in childbirth, which has been seen in the last 10 years, increasing for the first time in the past 50 years. The prenatal "vitamins" taken by nearly all pregnant women actually deplete our patients' vitamin C levels to a dangerous and life-threatening degree, thus contributing to clotting factor deficiencies and increased risk of hemorrhage, especially due to the "K" factor deficiency.

Because connective tissue strength is determined by the whole C molecule, C deficiency or taking ascorbic acid in standard prenatal "vitamins," which depletes your C levels, may also be a significant contributing factor to premature rupture of membranes, cervical incompetence, preterm labor and delivery, anemia, pelvic tissue weakness, stretch marks and more.

I used to recommend supplementing with berries as the most likely source of fruit-derived whole-food vitamin C. While this recommendation is still correct, I have discovered that they spray commercial berries with methyl bromide to stop mold growth. This bromine issue is extremely important as we discussed in Chapter 5 and 6 and could be a huge concern with regard to the development of breast, prostate, ovarian, thyroid and possibly pancreatic cancer.

So unless you grow or pick wild berries yourself, you do not know for sure what you are getting. To heat them is to kill them, so consume only fresh or frozen berries to get the whole-food C molecule. Heated jams, jellies and fruit pies, while absolutely delicious, deplete our vitamin C.

4. **Atherosclerotic plaque and vascular disease:** I may not be the first to suggest that vitamin C deficiency is the problem in plaque-forming vascular disease, but I might be one of the first to truly state what it means for these patients to be C deficient because of this ascorbic acid deception. The C molecule and copper utilization are responsible for the connective tissue strength and healing of every tissue in the human body. Without C (the real thing), the cells of our arterial walls do not hold together very well and they become leaky, especially near the heart where the pressures are the greatest. The healing response is to lay down a patch, or plaque, to stop the leaks. Cholesterol is not the issue in most cases.

The C molecule deficiency model as a cause of heart and vascular disease fits more accurately than any other theory thus far proposed. This concept is so simple and so important to our health that this change of awareness cannot happen fast enough. But first, physicians and nutrition leaders must recognize that ascorbic acid is not vitamin C, it depletes vitamin C from the body and it has numerous harmful effects, unlike the real C molecule. This is The Vitamin C Lie.

5. **Connective tissue weakness:** Joint, back, neck, knees, disks, cartilage, ligaments or tendons, fascia: Quite literally every piece of connective tissue in the human body requires the C molecule for its strength as well as the right concentrations of the minerals zinc and copper to be healthy. By the way, our connective tissue is supposed to be stronger than bone. This is not what we see. Copper cannot be utilized by the body and connective tissue cannot be formed correctly without the whole-food C molecule.

   Accordingly, nearly all back and neck disk degeneration, nearly every tendon rupture, nearly every knee ligament tear, nearly every hernia, every bulge, sag, droop, pinch and tissue "fall," nearly all pelvic relaxation from torn ligaments in childbirth, hemorrhoids, varicose veins, spider veins, loss of cartilage in joints leading to replacements and more orthopedic operations than we can imagine to the tune of billions of dollars, could all be most often prevented if we all had adequate whole-food vitamin C from early on in life.

6. **Type 1 hypothyroidism:** Thyroid hormone cannot be produced by the thyroid gland without the vitamin C molecule. Most type 1 hypothyroidism is probably related to chronic C deficiency. As we noted in Chapter 5, vitamin C regenerates selenoproteins essential for thryoid health, as well as facilitating copper utilization, both necessary for the formation of thyroid hormone. Therefore, the combination of C deficiency and selenium deficiency should be an exact recipe for developing type 1 hypothyroidism (failure of hormone production).

When we start to look at this vitamin C deception problem realistically, it becomes overwhelming in significance. I still cannot understand why it was allowed to happen. I suffered from it myself also for many years. I recognize the lack of awareness and the ignorance of some who argue that all we need is ascorbic acid.

From Dr. Thompson

I'll tell you a little personal story: Nine years ago, I fell during a "home improvement" project. I completely burst or exploded the bone of one vertebra, T9, and had a compression fracture of T12 and broke all the ribs in between. Doctors told me the chances were a million-to-one that I would ever walk again. I refused to accept that diagnosis because I knew some things they didn't. I had great faith and I had been taking whole-food C-complex for nearly four years by then. My disc tissue was so strong that it did not rupture. Even thought the bones were broken and had literally exploded, the discs remained intact.

My recovery was painful and slow, but I am fully functional, painfree and walking perfectly today. Walking is a blessing we so easily take for granted. In fact, I passed my military physical fitness tests, as part of my Army Reserve officer's status while on active duty in Operation Enduring Freedom, less than two years after the accident. I continue to thank my God with many prayers and in part credit the whole-food vitamin C complex for my complete recovery.

Vitamin D Hormone

This oil or "fat"-soluble vitamin (actually a hormone, not a vitamin) is also a complex substance with at least 10 different known compounds making up the D hormone molecule family referred to as D1, D2, D3, . . . , so it is important to get all the elements of vitamin D, not just one. D2 (ergocalciferol) is derived from plant sources. D3 (cholecalciferol) is derived from animal sources and is the form produced in the skin with direct sunlight. The vitamin D hormone complex is essential to proper mineral metabolism. If you remember the composition of bones and the mineral storehouse function of bones from chapters 2 and 3, it's important to add here that the vitamin D hormone helps in the movement of minerals in and out of the bones as they are needed elsewhere in the body. D is actually a hormone, not a vitamin per se. Deficiency should be corrected, but excess could be very harmful especially when the body already has an excess in intracellular calcium. We have to know for sure.

What else vitamin D hormone does:

- Monitors excretion of calcium through the urine and maintains proper blood calcium levels;

- Stimulates absorption of calcium and phosphorus from the intestines;

- Helps minerals harden bones;

- Helps maintain bone growth;

- Helps keep the nervous system healthy by regulating calcium levels in the blood;

- Plays a role in production and release of insulin to balance blood sugars;

- Works with parathyroid hormones to keep calcium at proper levels in the blood;

- Regulates cell growth and so may be protective against certain types of cancer;

- Regulates the permeability of cell membranes;

- Enhances immune function;

- Has a role in mood and depression;

- Contributes to muscle strength and helps regulate muscle tone.

- May prevent Type 1 diabetes.

Vitamin D hormone is a strange nutrient in that we get most of our supplies from sunshine on bare skin and from our HDL good cholesterol (the natural biochemical source of all our hormones). This isn't very practical in January in Alaska, where I live, or even if you live in New York, Illinois or Minnesota. Heck, Kathleen says it's a bad idea in the mountains of North Carolina where she lives. Fatty fish (think salmon and tuna) are the main food sources of vitamin D, but best if eaten as sushi or cold smoked or not heated. Cod liver oil is the huge winner on the vitamin D scale with an impressive 1360 IU per tablespoon. However, you need to avoid cod liver oil if your HTMA shows a calcium excess, or when your metabolic rate is slow for any reason. We have to know for sure.

We know that the body's ability to absorb vitamin D falls off as we age, and that deficiency can increase the risk of osteoporosis, some types of cancer, juvenile (type 1) diabetes, certain infections and multiple sclerosis. Studies estimate that 30 to 40 percent of elderly people with hip fractures are D deficient. (We guarantee 100 percent are mineral deficient.) Excess synthetic "vitamin" D, however, like the drug added to milk, can lead to excess calcium with the cascade of effects we already know about.

There is a vitamin D Lie, too, unfortunately, that comes from the notion that synthetic vitamin D hormone added to foods will make up for a shortfall. Synthetic vitamin D is like all the other so-called vitamins that are made from one element of a complex molecule. There has been a great deal of research on vitamin D recently and it is very promising, but we still don't know enough to take the risk of swallowing handfuls of supplements. In particular, synthetic vitamin D hormone added to homogenized cow's milk has been shown to cause adverse effects on heart, muscle and artery cell walls, probably because of the excess calcium. Worse yet, one study showed that infant formulas fortified with synthetic vitamin D had excessive amounts of this drug/imitation hormone vitamin.

The issue is how to get a dosage that will be sufficient without overdosing. Remember, "vitamin" D is really a hormone. As with any hormone, too much of the hormone can be just as bad as not enough, especially if your HTMA shows elevated intracellular calcium levels. Before you decide to take a vitamin D supplement, you need to know your calcium to magnesium ratios from a hair tissue mineral analysis (HTMA) and your overall tissue calcium levels. If you have an imbalance in your calcium/magnesium ratio, or a significant calcium excess in your tissues, vitamin D and cod liver oil may be harmful to you until you correct the imbalance. Taking this vitamin without knowing your levels, or taking it in large amounts, could greatly accelerate all the disease changes discussed in this book due to excess calcium. Your needs are also dependent upon your body fat levels because fatty tissues store up vitamin D. You should not take vitamin D unless you know you need it and you are paying careful attention to your intracellular calcium levels based on your HTMA results.

This one is really a no-brainer. You can get what you need from sunlight, free of charge, up to 10,000 IU per day. It doesn't take a lot and you don't have to worry about skin cancer if you keep your exposure time to 10 minutes for light-skinned people. Dark-skinned people need longer exposure time. Just go out in the sun with your face, head and arms uncovered, a couple of times a week at noontime and you'll be covered (pun intended). While our bodies can't store vitamin D for a very long period of time, this kind of exposure as often as you can do it will get you through most winters in the "lower 48" (an Alaskan term for everyone else in the U.S. except Hawaiian "islanders"), if you live south of a line from LA to Atlanta. In

Alaska, we've learned the value of fatty fish, halibut and salmon as sushi or cold smoked to help us get the vitamin D hormone we need to get through those long winters.

What is interesting is that the right sun exposure will correct D deficiency rapidly, but will not create an excess. Enough is enough. Our bodies stop producing the hormone vitamin D once we have enough, just like every other hormone when our bodies are functioning correctly. If we are taking D as a supplement, however, we can certainly get too much of this hormone. Synthetic D hormone toxicity from the drug form of the "vitamin" in humans has been reported with its related hypercalcemia (excessive blood calcium and intracellular tissue calcium), tissue calcifications, vascular disease, hypertension, stones, plaque, spurs and everything else we've mentioned in this book, including dementia and brain shrinkage. This does not happen with sunlight-produced natural forms of the vitamin. Enough is enough! Too much D hormone as well as not enough has been associated with disease and illness in humans. Know your level (I recommend between 40 and 60) and supplement correctly.

Vitamin E

Fat-soluble vitamin E is the subject of yet another of these endless lies. (Here's a simple mnemonic: "DEAK," D, E, A, and K are the fat-soluble vitamins, which must be taken with food). The Vitamin E Lie goes like this: We need the alpha-tocopherol in vitamin E as an antioxidant for protection against a variety of diseases of aging, including heart disease, cancer and diabetes. The Vitamin E Lie is similar to the vitamin C Lie in the sense that, much as ascorbic acid is only one part of the vast C-complex molecule, the alpha-tocopherol is only one piece of a large number of complex compounds that make up the vitamin E molecule. We need the whole intact molecule. Vitamin E:

- Is essential to reproductive health. Lab animals deprived of vitamin E were infertile;

- Is required for normal sexual development in both sexes;

- Is essential to the central nervous system, mental alertness;

- Is part of the endocrine gland system and has a role in thyroid, adrenal and pituitary glandular function, and magnesium utilization;

- Assists in controlling inflammation and repairing tissue damage;

- Participates in the maintenance of smooth skeletal and heart muscles;

- Is involved in iron absorption and the production of red blood cells;

- Contributes to skin and hair health;

- Contributes to kidney, liver and lung health;

- Has a role in blood-sugar metabolism;

- Has powerful antioxidant and free radical-taming properties and is important in regeneration of glutathione and the antioxidant properties of the vitamin C molecule;

- And much more.

Vitamin E is found in raw nuts, raw seeds, unrefined cold pressed vegetable and nut oils, wheat germ, flax seed meal, green leafy vegetables, broccoli, liver, alfalfa and corn.

So, back to the Vitamin E Lie: Like all vitamins, vitamin E is a complex molecule with many components. The main components are tocopherols and tocotrienols, but among these two main categories, there are eight known forms of tocopherols and four known forms of tocotrienols, four essential fatty acids, selenium, lipositols and xanthenes. This is the same story as with other vitamins: Making a pronouncement that just one piece of such a complex vitamin is *the* vitamin is plain and simple dishonesty and can be dangerous to your health.

"Natural" forms of the vitamin E complex when separated chemically from their parent molecule lose over 99 percent of their true potency and beneficial effects and may produce the same symptoms as the vitamin deficiency. This is called the "Reverse Effect" and is true not only for E, but also for A, C, D, K and to a lesser extent the purified forms of the B family. We must get the whole molecule to get the full benefit. All supposed adverse effects of the E vitamin are due to this error. The drug form "vitamin" E has adverse effects and lack of benefit in clinical research. The real E vitamin molecule has no known adverse effects and many known very important biochemical functions.

This is also why so many of the research studies on "vitamin E" have shown no effect or benefit and even possible harmful effects since researchers are using an inert drug, not the real vitamin E complex molecule.

For some inexplicable reason, the original study on the "vitamin" E isolate was a rat fertility study using alpha-tocopherol succinate. This study became the gold standard to determine how much of this substance was necessary to reverse infertility in rats fed a rancid diet. The naturally occurring vitamin E complex is a relatively stable molecule. The alpha-tocopherol has been shown to have the strongest antioxidant property of all the tocopherols in the vitamin E molecule.

In order to market the alpha-tocopherol as "vitamin" E, the supplement companies must use a stabilization process called "esterfication," which gives the product a long shelf life and prevents it from becoming rancid or oxidized. This process makes the alpha-tocopherol ineffective as an antioxidant in humans since it has been "processed." It is biochemically inert or inactive in humans. It works in rats, however, because they have different biological processes that can de-esterfy compounds. Therefore, the alpha-tocopherol as a succinate or an acetate molecule has no antioxidant or vitamin E effects in this form in humans.

What's more, in one study, vitamin E–deficient laboratory animals fed mixed tocopherols only died sooner than control animals who received no vitamin at all.

Another study, this one on humans, showed that a low concentration of vitamin E in the blood plasma was a greater risk factor for death from heart disease than was elevated cholesterol or high blood pressure. The E drug vitamin has also been shown to increase the risk of blood clotting, prostate cancer and has repeatedly shown lack of benefit. There should be some benefits if they were studying the right molecule. This should have been a clue, that scientists were testing a drug, not a vitamin. Yet, we need vitamin E to survive. What's the answer?

This one is simple, and cheap, too: Get your vitamin E from raw nuts and seeds, from unrefined cold-pressed vegetable oils or 100 percent whole-food vitamin E supplements.

Vitamin "F"—Essential Fatty Acids (EFAs)

OK. There is no such thing as vitamin F, although it is a name once attached to the need for the healthy fats we all need. Anyway, it fits neatly into our alphabet soup of vitamins and essential nutrients and it makes them easier to remember. We all need vitamin "F" (essential fatty acids) and, sadly, it is another part of The Vitamin Lie. We all need unsaturated fatty acids, sometimes called UFAs.

Yet sometime in the early 1980s, we as a nation got into a fat phobia. I'm not sure who started the idea that all fats are bad and that all fats make you fat. Nothing could be farther from the truth. However, we all started eating low-fat everything. Not coincidentally, we then started gaining weight. If you look at the graphs of the national obesity epidemic, its beginnings can be traced to exactly this same time period. We decided that it was OK to eat ice cream by the gallon, as long as it was low fat. Nothing slowed our national craving for French fries, and our intake of lethal trans-fatty acids went through the roof. We got supersized, literally. We are now dealing with a new "Generation XL."

We all need good fat in our diets. Without it, we die. Every one of the trillions of cell membranes in our bodies is predominantly composed of fat with protein molecules scattered over the inside and outside.

The key is we need the right fats, the UFAs that come from unrefined cold-pressed vegetable oils, raw nuts and seeds rich in linoleic and linolenic acids and the omega-3s that come primarily from deep water fatty fish and flaxseed.

Here's what UFAs do for you:

- Protect your heart by controlling cholesterol and triglyceride (blood fat) levels and minimizing disease-causing inflammation;

- Combine with cholesterol and protein to form the membranes that hold cells together;

- Help transport oxygen to all cells and tissues;

- Establish normal growth patterns in children;

- Improve mental and neurological health by easing depression and anxiety and enhancing attention and learning abilities;

- Keep brain cell communication healthy, reducing the risk of Alzheimer's disease. The brain is nearly 25 percent good HDL cholesterol. Low HDL cholesterol is associated with increased risk of Alzheimer's disease;

- Slow the course of arthritis and ease chronic pain and inflammation;

- Improve the course of pregnancy, promote healthy outcomes for the mother and long-term physical and mental health for her child;

- Promote healthy physical and mental development for our children;

- Enhance energy production;

- Produce hormones;

- Help insulate nerve fibers;

- Reduce the production of inflammation-causing prostaglandins;

- Lubricate skin, our largest organ.

The earliest sign of fatty deficiency is often dry, red, itchy skin and the onset of dermatitis and other skin diseases.

We get our vegetable-sourced UFAs from raw nuts and raw seeds and cold-pressed oils made from them. Most UFAs are destroyed by any heat over 160 degrees Fahrenheit, so roasted nuts and seeds and heat-processed oils are nutritionally without value and contain potentially toxic rancid fats. Check your labels carefully, because most oils are processed with heat and chemical solvents. The label should say your oil is cold pressed, unrefined or expeller processed, not cold "processed," which includes heat in the process as well as cooling.

We get omega-3s primarily from raw or cold-smoked fatty fish like salmon, tuna and cod. Omega-3 is also present to a somewhat less usable degree in flaxseed, some cold-pressed vegetable oils and green leafy, vegetables.

The omega-3s in fish oil are the most common source of these essential fats and two major elements are responsible for the health benefits:

- **DHA** (docosahexaenoic acid) has many positive effects, but perhaps the most impressive is its ability to help lower triglycerides. High triglycerides are linked to heart disease in most, but not all, research. Research also shows that DHA is important for helping pregnant women carry their babies to full term and gives their babies the maximum nourishment through breast milk, for visual and neurological development in infants, learning in young children, normalizing brain function, emotional and psychological well-being, preserving eyesight, insulin resistance (prediabetes and diabetes) and easing digestive and reproductive difficulties.

- **EPA** (eicosapentaenoic acid) is credited with reducing excessive blood clotting that can lead to heart disease. EPA also plays a role in reducing stress, keeping physical energy levels up, eye health and good brain function.

Alpha-linoleic acid, a third element of the omega-3s from plant sources, is converted to DHA and EPA in the human body, but the transition is inefficient, so it requires approximately ten times the vegetable-sourced omega-3s to receive the amount of DHA and EPA found in salmon, tuna or other cold-water fish, best eaten as unheated cold smoked or raw as in sushi to get the maximum fatty acid nutritional value.

Most fish oil products on the market are genuinely made from fish oil, so the composition of the product is not in question; it is the source and the processing that can be problematic. Mercury and heavy metal contamination are serious concerns for anyone who eats fish caught almost anywhere in the world. Wild-caught Alaska salmon is one of the few exceptions to this rule. Farmed fish are not worth your money because they are fed an unnatural diet that limits their omega-3 content and the farming methods include toxic chemicals that contaminate the fish as well as the ocean and even wild fish in the vicinity. We now also have GMO-farmed fish that raises additional concerns. There are supplements that are processed in such a way that they are safe and any heavy metal contamination is removed. Among them is Eicosamax (the ultrapure omega-3 product I recommend) and the shark liver oil product I highly recommend (Ocean Gold), but there are probably others as well. Molecularly distilled products also have a high degree of purity.

"Vitamin" GLA

Not really a vitamin, gamma-linolenic acid (GLA) is a fatty acid found in vegetable oils. Also called omega-6, it is found richly in safflower oil, evening primrose oil, black currant oil, borage oil and hemp seed oil. The human body produces GLA from linoleic acid. It has important anti-inflammatory effects and lacks the side effects of anti-inflammatory drugs. It may have benefits in atopic dermatitis (eczema), various immune disorders, arthritis and PMS, and in the treatment of some cancers it may have some potential to suppress tumor growth and metastasis. GLA is a building block for protein found in blood-clotting proteins and naturally existing calcium-binding proteins.

HDL Cholesterol (Vitamin "H")

The effects of HDL deficiency are huge with regard to hormone dysfunction, increased risk of Alzheimer's disease, as well as compromised immune systems and increased risk proven for stomach, lung and colon cancer. HDL cholesterol has also been shown to be protective against heart disease. Our brains are actually nearly 25 percent HDL cholesterol.

The yolk of an egg is pure HDL cholesterol, maybe our best food source of HDL. As long as the membrane surrounding the yolk is intact, the yolk is pure unoxidized healthy good HDL cholesterol. If that membrane is ruptured as the egg is heated for cooking (or scrambled), the yolk is exposed to oxygen, and thereby becomes a rancid fat that actually causes heart and vascular disease.

This is the simple truth about eggs: Never eat a scrambled egg yolk. Take out the yolk if you are baking. Eat the intact yolks frequently. We should call this The Egg Lie. We all need about between 4 and 8 intact egg yolks per week to get our necessary HDL good cholesterol. Our brains and hormones depend on it. How simple is that. HDL levels are best if over 70. We do not know if high levels are of any concern. Thus far, there have been no reports of high levels being associated with any disease. Low levels have been associated with a directly proportional increased risk of poor memory and Alzheimer's disease. It has been shown that the lower the HDL level, the greater the risk of all forms of dementia.

Vitamin K

Fat-soluble vitamin K was first identified as an antihemorrhagic compound in 1939, and called "koagulations" vitamin (Danish for coagulation spelled with a k). It is an integral part of the vitamin C molecule (the K factor). Vitamin K exists in two forms. The plant form (K1) phytomenadione is found in green leafy vegetables, spinach, turnip greens, dark lettuces, cabbage, cauliflower, brussel sprouts, peas, beans, egg yolk, tomatoes, potatoes and strawberries. This form of K participates in photosynthesis in plants.

The other natural form (K2) is menaquinone and is produced by gastrointestinal bacteria in humans and animals. The gastrointestinal bacterial production of the K2 Vitamin can be depleted when you take antibiotics.

Menadione is a synthetic form known as K3. High levels of the synthetic vitamin K3 can cause toxic reactions including increased red blood cell death and anemia. This synthetic form of the vitamin K3, commonly given to newborns, can also cause increased levels of bilirubin in the neonatal period.

Vitamin K also activates inactive fibrinogen to fibrin for blood clot formation. Vitamin K deficiency has been implicated as a risk factor for osteoporosis and it is known to interact with the vitamin D hormone and with calcium.

Breast-feeding is nature's way of building up healthy K2-forming bacteria in the neonatal gastrointestinal track. Breast milk actually contains over 10^3 gastrointestinal bacteria from the mother's gut (more than a UTI load of bacteria). These bacteria quickly populate the baby's gastrointestinal tract with healthy K2-producing bacteria.

The K factor in vitamin C is basically vitamin K. So once again we see the whole C molecule is critical for the vitamin K actions in the human. Vitamin K is also known to be synergistic with vitamin D hormone. In its natural form, it has no known toxicity or adverse effects. The synthetic form, vitamin K3, can cause biochemical disruptions and have adverse effects.

Finally. . .

I wish I could say to you, "Take this multi or this individual vitamin or that mineral formula." I can't. There are some very good products on the market, and some are even excellent. I hope to have some soon through my website.

It seems everyone has been deceived by thinking they need a women's formula, a men's formula, a prenatal formula or a children's formula. These products unfortunately always have various trace minerals added. If you already have an excess of any one of these minerals in your body, that supplement is bad for you. These minerals are obviously important and necessary, but must be given in the correct form and amount to meet your specific needs, not someone's idea of what *everyone* needs. It is my strong opinion that deficiencies and imbalances in vitamins and minerals are separate issues and should be addressed as such. They should never be combined into a one-size-fits-all.

Currently, there are very few vitamins that I can unequivocally recommend as the perfect product and none that can be considered the be-all and end-all of all products. I approach all supplements with the same caution and scrutiny that I use to evaluate and recommend medications. I want the best for my patients, the best for their needs and their budgets. But most importantly, I want what helps my patients get better and healthier. I remind my patients that their success in getting healthier is also my success. I can only be responsible for getting them on the best possible supplements for their long-term health; they have to be responsible for taking them consistently.

Whole-food is a very important key, as is balance. Know your balance and imbalance of minerals. Know your needs and excesses and eat as if your life and health depends on it. It does. Take a look at the resource section of this book and check in with us regularly at our website, www.calciumlie.com as we add new product recommendations and updates to the material in this book. We welcome reader recommendations through the website so we can expand our list of recommended products. To be sure, my patients don't have unlimited budgets for supplements and my standards are thus very strict for what I will and will not recommend.

Fast food does help our busy schedules at times, but consumers beware. I remind my patients that none of us are perfect and we can't expect ourselves to be perfect to improve our health. However, we must keep working at being healthy every day, and we must supplement correctly with the basics or our health will decline rapidly. Remember, little positive changes lead to bigger ones.

Taking the correct supplements is essential to maintain and improve our health. We can no longer rely on eating to be healthy. The essential balanced trace minerals and whole-food vitamins must be obtained consistently otherwise almost all other supplementation is futile.

I've said before that your results will be as good as your commitment to the dietary, mineral and vitamin program. If one good change is made, it will usually lead to two, then four, then more. I call this healthful congruence. Soon, life changes and you can really feel better than you ever expected possible, even if you think you are already healthy. We have to decide how well we want to age and keep working at it. Yes, you may make some mistakes, but never stop, even if some days are better than others.

POINTS TO REMEMBER

✔ A vitamin is a naturally occurring complex essential nutrient that the body either manufactures or derives from fresh food or other whole-food sources. A drug is a chemical compound that does not normally occur in the human body. Drugs are chemical substances synthesized or isolated by laboratories which may then be patented. Drugs may have some basis in naturally occurring nutrients and may even be marketed as "natural," but they have been synthetically or chemically altered or are merely fragments of the original substance. They may have effects, some good and some bad.

✔ Almost all "vitamin" supplements on the market today are actually drugs.

✔ All vitamins are complex molecules. Avoid any "supplements" that are made of only one ingredient or only a part of the whole-food molecule, e.g., so-called vitamin C that is composed exclusively of ascorbic acid. These are drugs, not vitamins, and they can be harmful or have drug-like effects, some good, some bad; but never make the mistake of thinking they are the same as the completely nontoxic real whole-food vitamin complex molecule.

✔ The multiple nutrient components that compose a vitamin molecule act synergistically, each enhancing the effects of the others.

✔ There are many medical myths about what each of the most common vitamins should be. Despite the depletion of our soils, it is still possible to get most of our essential vitamins from food, but this takes great care and is fraught with minefields and deceptions. Correct supplementation appears in my experience to be almost completely necessary to achieve optimal health. Your vitamins and supplements should all be made from vine- or tree-ripened whole-foods. End of story.

CHAPTER 8

Who Needs Calcium
and Why

A FTER PUBLISHING THE FIRST EDITION OF *The Calcium Lie*, it became clear to us that we left out an important piece of the puzzle. Most importantly, once again, we all need to know for sure *exactly* which minerals we need and why.

There is only about a 5 to 10 percent chance that you need more calcium. We need reliable HTMA results to tell for sure. There is a 100 percent chance you need minerals, so the story has not changed. The entire focus should be on knowing which minerals you really need, not on ones someone else thinks you need. The HTMA is how we tell.

I've been working with the HTMA information for more than 13 years and the relationship between those hair tissue mineral analysis results and my patients' health issues has become abundantly clear. While I often individualize the HTMA nutritional recommendations based on the most current health knowledge available, I have repeatedly seen outstanding results in applying this information. I avoid absolute conclusions about metabolism from the test, but I find the trends and physiologic relationship of the minerals to our long-term health scientifically reliable and reproducible.

Trace Elements, Inc. (TEI) of Houston, Texas, is still the only laboratory that I completely trust to give state-of-the-art reliable and accurate results for both the intracellular mineral levels and even more importantly the critical ratios that are most significantly responsible for, or a result of, our health issues and diet. I have no financial interest in TEI or any other company except my own medical practice. I use their HTMA service and recommend supplements from TEI when needed. I also recommend other very specific companies' products through my medical practice, and market these as such through my medical practice and online through Aurora Health and Nutrition (www.aurorahealthandnutrition.com).

I welcome the idea that more companies will start doing HTMA correctly, reliably and responsibly.

The trump card

I grew up playing cards as a social and family form of entertainment. Euchre was my favorite and still is, but hearts, spades and bridge were also common pastimes. We would spend hours playing games after meals. My grandfather was the best of all. He was physically handicapped, so sitting games or spectator sports like baseball were his favorites. My point here is that the game strategies and math I learned at my grandfather's card table apply quite accurately to the body's mineral physiology.

Calcium as it turns out is the king and most dominant mineral in our body's physiology. Its excess leads to the Calcium Cascade as we have described it in this book. There is, however, a calcium "trump," a physiologic response that rules over calcium. Whether you have this trump card in your personal physiology that rules over calcium is fairly unpredictable. It occurs in men about 4:1 over women, it is often associated with a "type A" personality, and this trump causes significant sodium retention and calcium and magnesium loss in the acute phase and both sodium and potassium retention in the chronic state, along with the same calcium and magnesium loss.

This trump card is stress.

For most of us, stress causes the adrenal glands to produce stress hormones 24/7. That is why this "trump" stress physiology is difficult to predict. Some individuals overproduce these adrenal hormones for both emotional and physical stress reasons. They were never intended to do so. Over time, this constant flood of stress hormones leads to chronic sodium retention. The only way to know for sure if you have this physiologic "trump" is through an HTMA result.

We all have stress in our lives. What is different about people who have this unfortunate trump card?

Adrenal hormone production is key to this equation. Remember the

Calcium Cascade? The suppression of adrenal hormones goes hand in hand with excess calcium intake, as the adrenal glands try to hold onto magnesium to balance the extra calcium. In these people, adrenal hormone production is reduced, therefore these individuals retain magnesium to compensate for their calcium and chronically lose sodium and potassium.

Adrenal hormone output, increase from stress or decrease from excess or relative excess calcium are key to both of these mineral profiles. Stress, however, creates a Catch-22 in which the increased adrenal hormones release causes the body to hold onto sodium and in turn lose calcium and magnesium. This is somewhat independent of calcium and vitamin D hormone intake due to the "trump." Calcium and magnesium loss are accelerated and this creates significant mineral imbalances. Over time, if the stress is chronic, the adrenal hormone overproduction-induced sodium retention will also lead to potassium retention. This apparently occurs so that water retention does not become extreme from a sodium/potassium imbalance.

This stress-related overproduction of adrenal hormone is gradually exhausting your adrenal glands and can cause many other mineral imbal-

---

Here's a little checklist that tells you if your stress levels are overtaxing your adrenals:

1. Are you a type A personality? Very competitive, self-critical, working long hours, always on the go?	YES	NO
2. Do you have high blood pressure?	YES	NO
3. Do you have heartburn and chronic indigestion?	YES	NO
4. Do you have chronic relationship issues, work-related issues, family issues or serious financial issues?	YES	NO
5. Do you have chronic illness or chronic pain issues?	YES	NO
6. Do you have trouble relaxing? ADD or ADHD (this includes children and adults)?	YES	NO

If you answered, "yes" to any of these questions, it's likely your adrenals are in overproduction mode caused by the acute or chronic stress issues and you may have serious mineral imbalances.

ances. It can cause your health to deteriorate at an alarming rate. Immune system compromise, hypertension, water retention, true gastric hyperacidity and more rapid aging all can be the results.

If you have chronic stress issues and you don't yet have high blood pressure, you're lucky. You can get on the bandwagon right now, make some simple changes and quite possibly save your own life.

I know I sound like a broken record, but it's so essential for all aspects of your health: Only an HTMA can tell us what is truly happening physiologically in your body. We must know for sure so you can begin to restore your health with a precise program of minerals and supplements and stress relief when needed.

Let's take a little time with biochemistry to look at how unrelieved chronic stress can cause your health to crash:

THE STRESS CASCADE (LEADING TO HIGH SODIUM LEVELS ON HTMA)

Stress leads to increased and near continuous adrenal hormone output and overproduction, excessive worrying, internalizing emotions; lack of tension relief is common,

and

Increased adrenal hormone output leads to sodium retention and magnesium loss,

and

Calcium is also lost through the kidneys as excess sodium is retained.

then

Chronic stress eventually leads to potassium retention

and

The result is true stomach hyperacidity, GERD, chronic esophagitis, chronic inflammation and related illnesses, reactive hypertension (elevated systolic more than diastolic blood pressure), chronic hypertension, increased risk of heart disease, accelerated aging and immune compromise issues including increased allergies and increased cancer risk over time.

It is critical for you and your doctor to identify these issues and to change their likely outcome. If you are chronically stressed, you may need serious sodium restriction in your diet. If the stress physiology is chronic and the potassium is also elevated, it is important to know that hypertension should never be treated with ACE inhibitors such as lisinopril or Zestril nor should it be treated with angiotension II receptor blockers such as Cozaar. The potassium retention caused by these medications could be fatal over time.

*Accurately identifying your place on this chart is the first step
to changing and potentially saving your life.*

So how do we treat stress? Diet and sodium restriction are at the core of treating stress. If the stress is long-term, you may also need to restrict your potassium intake or consumption of potassium-rich foods. Your doctor will need to correct the use of certain medications, most importantly ACE inhibitors if you have been taking them.

In this fairly uncommon situation, you will most likely need to *increase* your calcium intake from food and vitamin D hormone exposure from sunlight (or supplements where needed) along with balanced sea salt–derived trace minerals. Your HTMA will also probably tell us that you need more magnesium to help you restore the balance. Sea salt-derived trace minerals are about 30 percent magnesium plus all the other minerals we need. Adding magnesium alone may result in loose stools and takes away the benefit of all the other minerals in the sea salt–derived low-sodium mineral supplement and it is rarely ever needed.

Of course, managing your stress is the heart of restoring your balance of sodium as well as all the other minerals in your body and every other health aspect of your life.

When I have patients who are experiencing stress-related mineral imbalances, I ask them about stress relief activities. I hear all the typical answers on what they believe relieves their stress. Exercise is the most common answer, but prayer, meditation, sex, reading, yoga, changing work environment, changing relationships, counseling and drugs are all legitimate answers. But there is one simple activity that appears to be the most profound of all: walking 30 minutes every day. I am convinced that walking

---

Laura's Story

I remember Laura, a 60-year-old woman who came to me with complaints she was tired and had numerous aches and joint pain. Her HTMA showed that she had a classic stress pattern. Her HS-CRP blood test marker for significant cardiovascular inflammation in the heart muscle was at 30. That's 10 times the normal level! My prescription for her: Walk for 30 minutes a day. In just three months, without any other changes, her CRP levels dropped to 0.3—that was 100 times lower than it had been only 90 days earlier!

is the most significant of all stress-relief activities because it slows us down. Walking is also an amazing relationship builder. We all can benefit from a 30-minute walk daily to completely change the physiologic effects of stress on our health.

Kathleen has actually written a book on just this subject: *10 Best Ways to Manage Stress* (Take Charge Books, 2013). It's full of ideas about getting the stress monster under control.

Laura's story should be an inspiration to everyone to walk. Studies show that three 10-minute walks may be as effective as one 30-minute walk, so it's manageable even for the busiest lifestyle. Longer walks are OK, but they lead to quitting the activity more often, so I keep it to 30 minutes and make it part of my daily routine. You don't even have to walk fast; in fact, slower may be better. All you need is a sturdy pair of shoes, a rain poncho for rainy days, a warm jacket for winter and a wandering spirit. I promise: Regular walking will change your life. Walking at work does not seem to produce the same results, unless it is for stress relief. Many of my patients use treadmills. I am happy with that too. But the outdoors is magical sometimes. Keep walking as if your life depends on it. It does.

Another patient, Bill, was a retired high school PE teacher. He had been walking regularly for more than 25 years. As part of my evaluation, he had a CT heart scan performed with the finding of a very high calcium score, sometimes referred to as the "widow maker" because it supplies blood to nearly two-thirds of the heart.

I referred him to a cardiologist who performed an angiogram. This study revealed that he had a 95 percent obstruction of the left anterior descending artery, but walking had caused the development of collateral vessels, bypassing the obstruction and saving his life. A stent was not needed! What a great testimony for walking. The American Cardiology Society has determined that walking regularly for at least 42 minutes reduces the risk of heart disease.

Walking also helps build relationships, to an amazing degree. We become closer to those with whom we share our walks. It is cheaper and takes less time than counseling. I speculate that the reason the health benefits of walking are so profound is that it forces us to slow down. This may be why we get more stress relief from walking than from running. The pace of our lives dictates the need for rushing, running, planning, thinking, driving and stressing. Life is often hard. There are good times and difficult ones. Walking somehow seems to help us gain perspective.

I walk daily—rain, snow, ice, wind chill, dark, minus 25 degrees (remember, I live in Alaska!), no matter. Kathleen does, too. In fact, she wears a pedometer all the time and her day isn't over until she's hit the 10,000-step mark. Many days she exceeds the goal.

Both of us always walk outside. There is a soothing aspect to nature that cannot be duplicated on a treadmill or in a gym. We have fresh air here in Alaska where I live and so does Kathleen in her Blue Ridge Mountains. The beauty, wild animals (moose and caribou here), interesting plant life and the overall peace are all beyond compare. I am definitely packing a powerful gun during bear season to be sure. We do get grizzly bears in the area quite often. Kathleen doesn't pack a gun, but she does pack three large dogs for protection from the milder-mannered black bears on her trails.

I am convinced it is critical that you are completely comfortable, warm and dry on your walk. So get the right gear. Music and cell phone is fine as long as it does not interfere with your peace. When I feel rushed, I set the timer on the phone for 15 minutes and when it beeps, I turn around and return at the same slow pace. It is not exercise; it is stress relief—not to be confused. Walking on the beach barefoot also allows us to absorb minerals through our feet. I often encourage parents to rub the liquid ionic-balanced trace minerals into their children's feet at bedtime for just that reason. They love it and it improves their mineral content. We rarely do this barefoot thing in Alaska's chilly ocean waters, but we do walk on our beaches. Walking at work or just being on our feet for over 30 minutes is not the same.

POINTS TO REMEMBER

✔ Chronic (long-term) significant stress causes profound sodium and potassium retention leading to high intracellular levels and significant calcium and magnesium loss. This affects less than 10 percent of our population clinically. Sodium restriction is beneficial and often needed in these patients. Quite often, people whose HTMAs show stress patterns also have high blood pressure.

✔ All hypertension treatment recommendations for both medication use and diet changes (levels of sodium, potassium and calcium intake) need to be based on actual HTMA results. We have to know for sure exactly what the intracellular levels of sodium, potassium and calcium actually are and incorporate these findings into the treatment regimen.

✔ High sodium levels occur in a small minority of people with mineral imbalances and stress patterns shown on their HTMAs. This test is critical to identify these individuals.

✔ Acute (short-term) stress causes sodium retention first; intracellular potassium may not be affected early on or may even be low if the stress duration is not too long.

✔ In this minority of stress-induced mineral imbalances, I recommend increased dietary calcium intake (not through dairy products), adequate vitamin D hormone intake, balanced trace minerals and sometimes calcium supplements (like AlgaeCal, a sea-harvested plant material rich in calcium plus other sea salt–derived trace minerals). Walking should be recommended to almost everybody and especially for those with confirmed stress patterns. Walking has the most profound effect on reducing physical and mental stress on our bodies of all known stress-relieving activities. Thirty minutes a day, five or more times a week, is enough. It also builds and improves relationships and costs almost nothing.

✔ Stress management must be a regular part of a healthy life style.

CHAPTER 9

The Road Back to Health

S O NOW YOU'RE ARMED WITH A LARGE VOLUME of information and perhaps more biochemistry than you'd like. We've made it as painless as possible and only burdened you with what you absolutely need to know to take action. Your health is your most precious resource and your sole responsibility; it's a gift to cherish or to lose.

When we're facing the multitude of lies the medical and pharmaceutical industries have foisted on us, information is our best and only real weapon. You may have to read this book more than once, and underline and highlight in order to assimilate the information we have presented here. We realize it is complex and there is a lot. And yet, we keep trying to keep it as simple as possible. What we've offered you here is the best recipe we know to a path of better health.

In Latin, *docere*, the root word for doctor, also means "to teach." A good teacher always makes the complicated subjects seem easy to learn. We recognize that we have introduced many new concepts and paradigms as we connect the dots. Thus far, every single statement we have made has been scientifically confirmed or is already proven as fact.

There are several original contributions in this book, including the clear definition of:

- The five types of hypothyroidism

- The influences of Döbereiner's Triads in mineral physiology

- The refrigerator's influence on civilization's nutrition

- The importance of adequate mineral replacement in pregnancy

- The importance of HTMA in the treatment of hypertension and hypo-thyroidism

- The error in accepting a decline of bone mineral levels with aging

- The whistle blowing on The Calcium Lie in osteoporosis

- The influence of the whole-vitamin C molecule on heart disease and cholesterol metabolism

- And the Calcium Cascade and some of its consequences, just to name a few.

I urge you and your doctor to question what you think you know. I encourage my patients to be full partners with me in restoring their health. Their success is my success. As my patients improve their health through correct supplementation and mineral and hormone balancing, other people notice and ask what they are doing.

Now is the time for action. Don't wait another day. Health decline takes place gradually and over time for most of us. By the time you actually develop a disease or illness like hypertension, heart disease, cancer, diabetes or virtually any chronic disease, the triggers have probably been firing under the threshold of your awareness for some time, maybe even for years. The absence of a health crisis does not necessarily mean you are healthy.

This is your action plan to find your way back to health.

It won't happen instantly, although you'll probably notice some changes in a matter of days. Perhaps you'll feel more energy, or some simple symptoms, like dry skin or restless sleep or fatigue, will start to change for the better.

There will be bumps in the road, detours and days when you feel like all the effort isn't worth it. All we can say is, "Keep going."

I remember a sign I once saw that said, "When you're going through hell, keep on going." You *will* come out the other side and be healthier and stronger for the experience. If there is a little inconvenience along the way, it's a small price to pay for avoiding the major health problems that our society has come to associate with "normal" aging. I refuse to accept this.

I remind my patients that they do not have to be perfect to improve. I am not either. If they do not take all their supplements three times a day, every day, well, OK, neither do I. But most days, I do. If we keep taking steps forward every day, even small ones, these steps are still forward steps. We're not stagnated and we're not slipping backwards.

Don't wait and hope and keep your fingers crossed that you will remain healthy until the day you die. Few of us do. There are no guarantees in life, but I can assure you that committing to my program is definitely a step in the right direction.

I also encourage patients to show me all the supplements they have been taking. I inspect each and every one to see if it is potentially good, bad, not harmful or just plain damaging. Most of the time, I find my patients are wasting huge amounts of money on supplements that are not helpful, and many are harmful. The most common bad supplements contain drug vitamins and calcium or various incorrect mineral ratios. The key word in whole-food supplements is "food." Keep thinking of supplements as food that is helping supplement what is missing from our food. As Hippocrates once said, "Our food is our medicine."

It's possible to be vibrant and healthy when you're 20, 30, 40, 50 or far beyond. It is possible to be 60 or 70, 80 or even 90 and free from heart disease, diabetes, dementia, cancer, cataracts and canes. It is never too late to start. I have 60-, 70- and even 80-year-old patients beginning this program and loving it. At the beginning, your road back to health will take some extra focus, but it will become second nature within weeks. Your goal should be to maintain optimal or improved health as you age. Intellect, eyesight and mobility should be our anti-aging priorities.

Take it a day at a time and do what you can. It definitely is easier and requires fewer supplements to maintain our health than to restore it. Prevention has always been shown to cost less, no matter what.

Little changes can make big differences. You had to learn to crawl before you could stand, stand before you could walk and walk before you could run. You probably fell down a few thousand times at first. Insanity is to keep doing the same thing and expecting different results. Improve one thing and you will improve two, two and you will improve four. Getting healthier soon becomes a congruent lifestyle.

If you only follow this program and improve one meal a day, you'll be 33 percent successful. That's highly significant in scientific terms. If you do what I am asking for two meals a day, that is a 66 percent success rate.

That's off the charts in terms of what scientists gauge as great results and you *will* get those kinds of changes if you stay with the program. If you adopt this plan as your complete lifestyle and adhere to it 99 percent of the time, your results will be beyond your imagination. I'm living proof of this, as are many of my patients.

Food is still the foundation

The great news: A very significant part of your road back to health will come from eating the right foods. You can get most of your necessary nutrients—vitamins and minerals—from food. Choose the right foods, according to your hair tissue mineral analysis (HTMA) results and its specific food recommendations, then your return to health will be far less expensive in economic terms than if you rely entirely on supplements.

This may seem like a contradiction of our earlier statements, but despite the depletion of our soils, food is still the best source of unrefined carbohydrates, protein, and sometimes vitamins (when they are made from vine-ripened foods grown in soil not depleted of its mineral content), sometimes minerals and many of the other nutrients we need. Humans cannot live on supplements alone, no matter how high the quality!

Based on our current food-growing and marketing practices, I believe supplements are essential, and we especially need minerals and the whole-food C vitamin.

As much as possible, eat vine-ripened, locally grown organic foods. You'll still have to add supplements, but this will give you the best possible sources of vitamins and minerals from your food.

Go organic as much as your budget will allow. You can find a list of the Dirty Dozen, the foods most often contaminated with pesticides and herbicides, at: http://www.ewg.org/foodnews/. I'd definitely add any members of the squash family to that list because they have been shown to have concentrated organophosphates, highly toxic pesticides and herbicides.

Buy locally produced foods when they are available because their nutrient content will probably be higher. Don't let the lack of a budget for organic foods or locally available produce be a stumbling block for you. Do what you can. Anything you do will help your body.

Start to think of food as the best possible nourishment for your body.

Here are a few great ways to get your vitamins through whole-food:

- Eat at least one-half an orange every day for whole-food vitamin C, or blend it with fiber, rice bran and fresh frozen raspberries (my favorite) or fresh frozen rose hips (these are very plentiful in Alaska). I usually limit fruit intake to about 6 ounces per day. More than that is simply too much sugar, even when it is natural fruit sugar.

- Beware of fruits, especially berries, which are often sprayed with bromine to stop mold from growing, which does not have to be included even on organic labels. Please be sure you are on enough iodine (at least 12.5 mg per day) to counteract this cancer-causing mineral.

- Enjoy one-fourth cup of raw pumpkin and sunflower seeds for essential fats, vitamin E and numerous B vitamins. Mix your seeds with organic raisins or cranraisins for vitamin C and potassium.

- Supplement with at least one tablespoon of stabilized rice bran powder every day. Rice bran contains more than 72 nutrients. It is high in B1, B3 and B6 in the whole-food form and with more than 2 grams of fiber per serving. I think the food value of stabilized rice bran is worth over $1,000 in store-bought supplements for around $5 at our local grocery.

- Eat as many vegetables as possible every day (not including high glycemic index veggies like potatoes, corn and peas) and vary the types of fruits and vegetables you eat. Minimize the amounts of fruit you eat and maximize your vegetables. Try to make vegetables at least 40 percent of your total food intake.

- Use unrefined, unprocessed sea salt or rock salt liberally if it is determined by reliable HTMA that you are in the 90 percent who need it. Remember, this type of salt contains all the ionizing minerals including iodine (not just sodium chloride) and in the perfect proportions. Table salt has no nutritional value at all.

   While this type of diet may not give you every single nutrient you need, it will go a long way toward promoting the best health you can achieve.

Anything you put in your body should be dedicated to your return to health. This is what I call healthful congruence.

   Fresh foods are almost always best, although there is some argument in favor of frozen foods, which are picked at the peak of their ripeness and quickly preserved by freezing. Avoid canned foods except tomatoes and beans. The high heat in the canning process destroys nearly all vitamins and minerals in foods, and the cans can be the sources of toxic minerals like tin and aluminum, so choose foods preserved in glass jars. Tomatoes and beans may be a necessary exception to this rule. Certain vitamins and fiber are actually released during the cooking and canning processes for these foods.

Avoid pasteurized foods as much as possible, since the heating process of pasteurization destroys enzymes, vitamins and nutrients. Hopefully, the governments and the people of the world will demand cold pasteurization done with electron beams (special light).

Most foods are best eaten raw or cooked very lightly. Steam or lightly sauté, bake or broil foods.

Avoid the microwave like the plague! Microwaves destroy most of the nutrient value in foods and make them worthless. Portuguese researchers found that broccoli zapped in the microwave with a little water lost 97 percent of its antioxidants, while lightly steamed broccoli only lost 11 percent.

Best, yet, eat the major proportion of your fruits, vegetables, nuts and seeds raw.

I love the idea of pulverizing raw vegetables in a high-speed blender. This soup (never heated above 110 degrees Fahrenheit or better yet, not heated at all) offers our bodies the most absorbable nutrients possible. Add a little organic chicken broth, a clove or two of garlic, a dash of cayenne and it's a delicious quick healthy meal in a glass.

I don't recommend juicers. They take out the fiber, which is a very important part of our diet. Always eat fruit 30 minutes before or two hours after protein and never eat it with a regular meal or from a jar or can.

Shop often and buy small amounts so you'll have the freshest possible foods on hand. The longer a food remains in the refrigerator, the more nutrients it loses.

If you have the space and the inclination, grow some of your own food. Every little bit helps. You have complete control over the garden and you can keep toxic chemicals out, even if you have to sacrifice a small percentage to the birds and the bees and other critters. Even a tomato plant on an urban balcony or a jar of alfalfa sprouts on a New York apartment window can serve as an inspiration to keep your feet on the road to health. There are few greater pleasures on this earth than biting into a sun-warmed tomato you just harvested from the garden you planted with your own hands.

Take some time to savor and appreciate your food. There was actually a study of prisoners fed a really terrible diet of prison food. Those who gave thanks for their food, in whatever spiritual tradition they preferred, actually gained more nourishment from that food and had far fewer physical illnesses than those who simply chowed down.

And speaking of chowing down, do take time with your meals and chew your food thoroughly. Chewing and mixing your food with the digestive enzymes in saliva while it is still in your mouth is the first part of the digestive process. If you are swallowing large chunks of barely chewed food, you'll gain little nourishment from it. Think of your mouth as that high-speed blender and pulverize your food into small pieces so you can get the maximum nutritional value from it.

Also, as a general rule, don't drink with your meals; drink before or two hours after. This extra fluid may dilute your digestive enzymes and decrease your ability to digest your food completely.

Getting started

Here's the most important first step: Get a hair tissue mineral analysis (HTMA). This is really the only way you can determine your exact mineral status and from that, learn what you need to do to improve your health and prevent medical problems from developing. In my experience, it may be the most important health test that exists. It is the foundation for everything I have been talking about throughout this book. Only when you and your doctor know for sure your mineral status and important ratios can you begin the journey back to health with the right diet, minerals and supplements for your unique situation.

I've said before, the only laboratory that I recommend for an accurate HTMA is Dr. David Watts' Trace Elements Inc. in Addison, Texas. This lab adheres to the highest possible standards and I absolutely trust their results.

Dr. Watts is a brilliant scientist whose database of more than 1,000,000 HTMA results shows distinct mineral patterns associated with various medical problems, imbalances and deficiencies, and tissue levels of key toxic minerals. This extensive data pool gives scientific validation to the links between mineral deficiencies and imbalances and manifestations of disease, ranging from high blood pressure to osteoporosis, thyroid function, adrenal function and more.

You need to get an HTMA from Trace Elements Inc. through a HTMA healthcare provider who uses this lab, since Trace Elements, Inc., will only accept samples submitted by physicians. The report will be much more meaningful with the help of a healthcare professional trained and experienced in the interpretation and application of the results. Your healthcare practitioner should guide you in the correct ways to address imbalances and to begin to reverse and correct disease trends.

Correct collection of the hair sample for the HTMA is a must. Please carefully follow the collection directions so you'll get accurate results.

Six important steps on the road back

Here are six steps I consider most essential for good nutrition. Do these and you'll be well on the road to great health and long life.

1. Drink pure water

Water is the stuff of life. Most of us need more than we drink. Everyone needs at least 64 ounces of water a day, more if you are overweight, a heavy exerciser or live in a very warm climate. As a general rule, we need to drink one-half of our body weight in ounces of water daily. For example, if you weigh 150 pounds you would need to drink 75 ounces of water daily, or two and one half quarts of pure water every day. Remember 72 percent of your body's weight is water and you need to keep that balance in order to be healthy.

Water helps sweep toxins from your body.

Get the purest water you can. If you have municipal drinking water, consider buying a good quality filter. These can cost anywhere from $200 for a quality countertop filter to $3,000 for a whole-house filter. As a general rule, filters that have a carbon block filter that is changeable put glue in the water because the carbon is glued into a carbon block to hold it into the filter. I recommend pressed carbon block without glue. See the Resources section for my recommendations of the best water filters or www.calciumlie.com.

This topic is hugely complicated. Take your time and have your water tested to identify your specific water needs carefully. Your life depends on it.

I am convinced that drinking alkaline water may be a good idea. Although there is little science to support it, the concept makes sense. We know that too much sugar intake (especially as fructose) and insulin resistance creates an acidic condition in the human body called acidosis. We know acidosis increases cancer risk. It makes sense that drinking alkaline water could be good idea to neutralize the typically acidic human body. You can buy whole-house water alkalinizers for around $1,000.

Avoid bottled water since much of it is little more than tap water put in a plastic bottle that will expose you to xenoestrogens, hormone disruptors that leach from the plastics. Plastic bottles are also environmentally unfriendly and extremely overpriced. For the same reason, drink all of your water from glass containers. If that is impossible when you are traveling, buy a stainless-steel water bottle and carry filtered water from home or take a filter with you on your trip.

Never drink distilled water, which has had virtually all nutrients and the very life of it removed. To do so also increases your need for the minerals that are naturally present in good quality water.

And think of the water you bathe in. Your skin is the body's largest organ and it absorbs toxins or nutrients. If you are showering in chlorinated water, the warm water opens your pores and your body literally drinks in the chlorine and other contaminants and brings them into your body. Ditto for hot tubs. Definitely stop using bromine-containing additives if you have a hot tub. Go back to chlorine. It is less toxic than bromine, it interferes less with iodine in our bodies, and it evaporates or dissipates out of the hot tub and out of your body more readily. If you shower before you enter the hot tub and use natural filtration systems, you'll need very little chlorine. Even better, sea salt-water hot tubs with ozone purification and ultraviolet water sterilization technology would be best. If a whole-house water filter isn't in your budget, you can buy an inexpensive shower filter that will cost you less than $10.

2. Take ionic sea salt–derived minerals

In nearly 2,000 patients I have tested in my practice, there has been only one person who had a near-perfect mineral balance. (It wasn't me!)

We all need minerals and virtually none of us get enough. Ionic minerals are the only ones that are completely available for our bodies to use because they are water-soluble and they naturally carry an electrical charge that allows them to be carried through the cell membranes.

Besides the trillions of functions they perform in our bodies, these minerals are the transport system for vitamins and amino acids into our cells. Without adequate minerals and without minerals in balance, these nutrients can't get into our cells and our bodies simply won't function as they should.

See the resource section for my recommendations on ionic mineral supplements. Sadly, there aren't very many I can recommend in good conscience. I'm always looking for more quality recommendations, so if you know of high quality ionic sea salt–derived mineral products or 100 percent whole-food vitamins, please contact me via my medical office or website, www.calciumlie.com.

The best source of ionic minerals is in unrefined sea salt and rock salt, if your HTMA shows you do not have a sodium excess associated with stress as explained in Chapter 8. If you are deficient in sodium, add harvested pure sea salt liberally to your foods and forget the myth about salt causing high blood pressure. That's nonsense for 90 percent of us! We have to know for sure. High blood pressure is more likely caused or contributed to by a combination of excess calcium, low intracellular sodium levels and intracellular amino acid deficiencies, as we discussed at length in Chapters 2, 3 and 4.

I'm not tooting my own horn when I tell you that the only ionic sea salt–derived trace mineral supplement for the 90 percent of us with low potassium I have found is sold only through my office and on my website. I am not being greedy here; it's just that I was fortunately able to convince the manufacturer to formulate the product exactly according to my specifications. I know it works! All sea salt-derived trace mineral products are good for everyone; however, the one I recommend is also corrective for the low intracellular potassium levels so often associated with calcium excess.

I recommend a minimum of 3 grams per day of trace minerals (6 tablets or $1^1/_2$ teaspoons of the liquid form). I remind my patients that water and minerals are the two most important substances we must put into our bodies every day. I encourage patients to take minerals with every glass of water and meals to maximize their intake and correct and prevent further deficiencies.

3. Whole-food vitamins

Almost all of us need supplements because we simply aren't getting our full complement of vitamins and minerals from our food. Eating to be healthy is probably no longer practically possible. We must supplement with food-derived nutrients and minerals. Unfortunately in our fast food nation, eating to be unhealthy is common and simple since it requires very little effort.

Almost all of us need additional supplements to help correct imbalances and deficiencies and to help prevent and treat specific disease conditions.

Avoid vitamins made from anything but 100 percent organic whole-foods that have been vine ripened. Unless you have a specific purpose for taking those store-bought vitamins that are actually drugs, they will not help you and they can potentially harm you. I use them short term in specific circumstances to achieve mineral balance according to the HTMA results. But I do not compromise on the whole-food vitamin C and E requirements.

As we have discussed throughout this book, essential whole-food vitamins are the only way to ensure you will get all of the complex molecular elements contained in these nutrients. You need all of the nutrient components together in their whole-food form to get the full benefits of these molecules.

Some vitamins have dozens, and possibly even hundreds, of specific nutritional components. We may not even know about some of them yet, since more and more are being discovered every year. We do know that many of these elements work synergistically, meaning that they enhance one another's effectiveness, which is the best argument I can think of for 100 percent whole-food vitamins that contain all the components with which foods were designed.

We have the same problem in recommending whole-food vitamins since there are so few on the market and many false or misleading claims are made. Check the resource section of this book and check in frequently on our website, www.calciumlie.com. We'll be adding new information as it is available and when I hear about new products that I can in good conscience recommend.

I currently only recommend Innate pure whole-food vitamins, especially their vitamin C and Vitamin Only™. I also recommend the Unique E whole-food vitamin E, as these are the only products that I can confirm are 100 percent whole-food. As I said a couple of paragraphs back, these whole food multivitamins and corrective trace minerals were formulated to my specifications uniquely for me, so they are only available through my office and my website, www.aurorahealthandnutrition.com.

The best natural sources of readily available vitamins include raw seeds and stabilized rice bran powder. Raw seeds have all known B complex vitamins (remember there are more than 50 of them), E complex and essential fatty acids. Also eat dried, frozen or vine-ripened fresh fruit and berries to get vitamin C complex in its whole-food form. Almost all store-bought fruits and vegetables are not vine ripened and, therefore, they have little mineral content and virtually no vitamins. Using the correct form of nutritional supplements can reap huge long-term benefits.

4. Essential fatty acids

The correct form of essential fat is vital to human health. And yes, it is time for an "oil change in our thinking." There are good-for-us saturated fats and good-for-us cholesterol. There are bad-for-us rancid oxidized and trans-fatty acids. Every cell membrane in the human body is composed largely of essential fatty acids. Having too much of the wrong kind of fat can cause a host of adverse health issues. It is the variety and quality of the fatty acid intake that is most important. Too much of one kind of fat can lead to trouble.

When The Fat Lie made us paranoid that fat would make us fat, we derailed our nutrition and actually triggered weight gain. The historic obesity charts released by the Centers for Disease Control and Prevention substantiate that the beginning of the low-fat diet craze in the early 1980s corresponds exactly to the upward trend in obesity in the United States.

Get your essential fats from the best possible food sources. There are two essential fatty acids that we need: omega-3 in the form of alpha-linolenic acid, or ALA, and omega-6 in the form of gamma-linoleic acid, or GLA. These two are considered essential because humans can't manufacture them within our bodies.

5. Eat raw nuts and/or seeds daily

They are excellent sources of essential fats—the good kind that you need

A little fat chemistry
(Skip this if it sounds too complicated)

Fatty acids are glycerol molecules with one, two or three fatty acids attached. Lipid bio-chemistry names these compounds based on the number of carbon atoms and the degree of saturation (that is, how many hydrogen atoms are bonded to the carbon atoms). They are classified as long chains (over 14 carbon atoms), medium chains (8 to 12 carbon atoms) and short chains (2 to 6 carbon atoms). In general, medium-chain unsaturated fatty acids are the best for human health.

Every cell membrane in our body is mostly made up of essential fatty acids arranged in layers and connected like chains, with protein molecules interspersed on either side of the membrane. Having too much of the wrong kind of fat can cause a host of adverse health issues. It is the variety and quality of the fatty acid intake that is most important. An over-abundance of one kind of fat or an obstruction of their metabolism (as with vitamin C defi-ciency and elevated cholesterol) can lead to adverse effects.

In general, omega-3 fatty acids make good things in the body and is the most important. They are the building blocks of hormone-like substances called prostaglandins. Omega-6 tends to form the inflammatory prostaglandins which do have a purpose, but less is better. Medium-chain-length fatty acids such as C8, C10 and especially C12 may have the greatest health benefits. These are found in mother's breast milk, saw palmetto, bitter melon, and are a minor component of extra virgin cold-pressed coconut oil.

every day. In 2003, the FDA approved the following health claim for seven kinds of nuts:

> "Scientific evidence suggests but does not prove that eating 1.5 oz per day of most raw nuts as part of a diet low in saturated fat and choles-terol may reduce the risk of heart disease."

However, if those nuts are roasted, they lose almost all their nutritional value and become toxic, oxidized, rancid fat like you find in virtually all store-bought peanut butter. Always opt for raw nuts and seeds. In any case, limit your intake to not more than 2 ounces daily. (We know it's hard to stop once you start popping those delicious raw cashews or almonds.) How-ever, if you are above your ideal body weight, opt for raw seeds only, and skip the nuts. The nuts have too much fat and will almost always keep you from losing weight.

I only eat peanut butter made at home from raw nuts, sea salt and a tiny amount of extra virgin olive oil. It must be refrigerated in an airtight container to keep it fresh. It is delicious and can be made from various kinds of raw nuts. Beware however of mold issues, especially with raw peanuts.

Raw pumpkin seeds are particularly good sources of essential fats as well as zinc, iron, calcium and phosphorus, with some magnesium and copper. There is a mix of complex vitamin E and B vitamins, with whole-food niacin being the richest in pumpkin seeds and rice bran powder. Pumpkin seeds are also rich in the essential amino acid methionine.

Sunflower seeds are also very high in potassium, low in sodium, with healthy levels of zinc, iron, calcium, copper, manganese and phosphorus. They also have substantial levels of the essential amino acid methionine, which helps to detoxify the body, activate enzymes and improve cellular energy production.

Raw sunflower seeds are rich in B-complex vitamins and one of the few naturally occurring food sources of vitamin D. Always opt for raw seeds and limit your intake to 1/4 cup daily. Those individuals with a high tissue copper level based on HTMA results should temporarily avoid these seeds and opt for pumpkin seeds instead.

Most nuts, including almonds, are also high in copper, so don't eat them unless your HTMA confirms you need the copper. Almost all ADD and ADHD in children and adults is associated with high copper levels and can be reversed with correction of this imbalance. Our bodies cannot utilize copper without the whole-food vitamin C molecule. Thus, copper accumulation is often a sign of vitamin C deficiency due to poor copper utilization.

Use only expeller-produced cold-pressed oils made from nuts and seeds. This means use extra virgin olive oil, sesame oil or cold-pressed virgin coconut oil only. Heat processing and cooking generally destroy the delicate structures of the fat molecules, rendering them virtually void of nutritional benefits. After heating, the fats become rancid and toxic. We all know what bad oil can do to our cars; our bodies are the most important cars we drive. Treat yours well. Put the best possible oils in it. Avoid "cold-processed" oils. This is a marketing gimmick and deceptive, and means they were cooled somewhere along the process. Good quality cold-pressed oils will indicate on their packaging that they have been processed without any heat or chemicals.

Get healthy fats from fresh-caught wild cold-water fatty fish like salmon, halibut and tuna. Eat them at least once a week; twice a week is better if you're sure they come from a mercury-free source. If you're not sure, ask. There is no equal to fresh Alaska wild salmon or halibut. Sushi or cold smoking is truly the best way to receive these omega-3 fatty acids that cooking essentially destroys. Raw fish needs to be handled very carefully to avoid bacterial contamination. Parasites are also a common concern with raw fish, but they are easily treated.

Egg yolks are a great source of good-for-us HDL cholesterol except when scrambled, which oxidizes the good cholesterol. We've discussed this in detail in previous chapters.

6. Eat high-quality proteins

The protein we humans get in our diets primarily come from meats, seafood, eggs, beans, chicken, game meat, duck and turkey. These protein sources are the source of the essential amino acids that are the building blocks of every protein molecule, hormone, neurotransmitter, cell membranes and immune molecules. They are important to the biologic function of every cell in the human body.

We must get these amino acids from proteins we eat every day, since we cannot store them for later use.

A shortfall of just one of the 10 essential amino acids can result in deterioration of the proteins inside the body. Your body will actually "rob" amino acids from muscle tissue to make up for a shortfall, which is a potential problem with some very low calorie diets.

These 10 essential amino acids are necessary for critical body functions, and there are at least a dozen or more additional amino acids that play vital roles in human nutrition and metabolism.

Essential amino acids are phenylalanine, valine, arginine, threonine, tryptophan, isoleucine, methionine, histidine, leucine and lysine. The other most important amino acids are cysteine, glycine, glutamine and tyrosine. (See Chapter 4 for details about the amino acids.)

Our primary sources of amino acids are meats, seafood and eggs, which contain all of the amino acids necessary for our survival. Eggs, in fact, are the protein source that is the most similar to human protein of all known food sources.

Proteins can also be obtained from grains, sprouted grains, raw nuts and raw seeds. Vegetarians, particularly vegans who do not eat any animal protein, must pay close attention to combining protein sources so that the full complement of amino acids is part of their diet every day. For example, a homemade raw peanut butter sandwich on a sprouted grain bread such as Ezekiel bread, black beans and brown rice or a bean burrito made with a sprouted grain tortilla would make a complete protein meal with all the essential amino acids. Unfortunately, vegans and vegetarians commonly suffer from severe mineral deficiencies and generally lose digestive enzyme capabilities over time.

Choose your meats, seafood and eggs carefully. When at all possible, buy organic meats and poultry that have been produced without antibiotics or added hormones or choose game meat.

Buy only wild-caught seafood from cold waters where heavy metal pollution is diminished. Seafood is a good source of protein and essential fats, but farmed seafood comes from a toxic soup. Avoid it at all costs.

Be careful not to mix fruit and protein in the same meal, which causes the protein to ferment in the gastrointestinal tract, releasing alcohol into the bloodstream and causing yeast overgrowth in the intestines and, in some cases, in the bloodstream. This is considered a "bad food combination." Fruit should be consumed one-half hour before or two hours after eating protein.

For most of my patients, I recommend avoiding or minimizing dairy products, since dairy products are high in calcium, and since most of us have calcium excess, we don't need these calcium-rich foods.

7. Get essential monosaccharides

This is probably a new recommendation for most of you and is a subject for another book, so bear with us while we enter some uncharted territory. Every protein molecule in the human body is dependent on monosaccharides for its action(s). Monosaccharides, the simplest form of carbohydrate molecules found in the body, are absorbed through the intestinal wall and carried in the bloodstream to tissues where they may be stored or used, in some cases, as an energy source.

On the biologically active end of every protein molecule is a complex monosaccharide receptor. These receptors are quite literally the keys that unlock every biochemical reaction in the human body, ranging from the formation of DNA and RNA to blood type, the creation and action of insulin, the action of all hormones, and every cell membrane receptor. Without the monosaccharide keys and the correctly fitting monosaccharide locks, things just don't work.

Monosaccharide deficiencies are implicated in nearly all abnormal autoimmune responses whereby immune molecules, called immunoglobulins, become abnormal immunoglobulins. This takes place when there is a nutritional deficiency of monosacharides and a substitution of a monosaccharide on the key or lock is made with the wrong monosaccharide. These immune molecules literally pile up because they can't find a receptor to bind to. The key literally doesn't fit the lock.

Eventually, these protein molecules with dysfunctional receptors accumulate, triggering an immune response. These proteins then become foreign proteins triggering an autoimmune or allergic reaction in the body. This process then causes the immune system to attack these molecules and/or normal healthy tissues. Specific monosaccharide deficiencies and substitutions have been shown to be a factor in several autoimmune diseases such as systemic lupus erythematosus, rheumatoid arthritis, juvenile rheumatoid arthritis, ankylosing spondylitis, scleroderma and Sjogren's syndrome.

In one study, patients with autoimmune diseases were compared to matched controls of patients without the diseases. Each of the autoimmune diseases in that study was found to have specific deletions and/or substitutions of at least one specific monosaccharide on a specific immunoglobulin protein molecule receptor that was exactly the same in all affected patients, with a huge statistical significance. The medical profession has largely ignored this data because it didn't make sense or lead to a drug therapy. After all, their current way of thinking is if you have one of these illnesses, you couldn't possibly have a nutritionally derived illness, so you must have a steroid or drug deficiency. This is, of course, completely illogical. But this is the core treatment regimen for most exacerbating autoimmune diseases.

It seems hard to believe that one simple sugar molecule could make that much difference or create that much havoc in the human body.

Remember that the entire difference between blood types A, B, AB and O is only one simple monosaccharide molecule on the terminal monosaccharide receptor that specifies your blood type. We long ago recognized what happens if you receive a transfusion of the wrong blood type, especially a second time. It will potentially kill you. This creates a whole new perspective about the significance of monosaccharide deficiency, imbalance and substitutions on our protein molecules.

The nutritional lack of these substances coupled with our decreased ability to synthesize these molecules as we age further complicates the problem. These monosaccharide deficiencies are preventable. A teaspoon of maple syrup every day in your oatmeal or fruit smoothie is a good way to add at least four of these essential monosacharides.

Between the ages of 20 and 60, our bodies lose 70 percent of our receptor protein activity, due to the gradual depletion of the number of monosaccharide receptors on the ends of each and every protein molecule in our bodies. This causes our biochemical reactions to run less efficiently. It is like changing from a jumbo jet to a two-cycle gas engine. Both engines work, but one is 70 percent efficient, the other is around 30 percent efficient. Which would you rather have flying your airplane?

When we're young, we are more likely to have sufficient enzymes and substrate or fuel, and cofactors to complete the nearly 16 steps it takes to convert the more complex sugars into the various other monosaccharides, such as the conversion of glucose to fucose. As we age, this process becomes less efficient and is no longer driven to completion. Healing becomes slower; hormones become less efficient and, in some cases, immune diseases such as cancer and autoimmune diseases such as lupus and diabetes may develop because our immune responses and cell membranes lack the correct receptors (the keys and locks don't fit).

Monosaccharides are divided into six major types of sugar molecules: glucose and its derivative N-acetyl glucosamine, galactose and its derivative N-acetyl galactosamine and four lesser-known sugars: fucose, xylose, acarbose and manose. For the most part, they do not occur in our diets. For our purposes in this book, there are very few good natural food sources of monosaccharides, but you will find some of them in some fruits, berries, melon and in some root vegetables like sweet potatoes, parsnips, beets and onions. They're also in honey and pure maple syrup and most other tree-sap syrups. I believe tree-sap syrup (pure organic maple syrup) is the best source for the money.

You don't need to eat large amounts of these foods to get the monosaccharides you need. A handful of strawberries, half a small sweet potato, a fresh onion on your burger or a teaspoon of maple syrup in your morning oatmeal should do the job quite nicely for most people under 40.

They are also available in a supplement form and, if you're over 40 or have autoimmune disease, I think it's a good idea to include these in your supplement regimen. If you're over 60 or if you have any type of autoimmune disease, you really need to add monosaccharides.

See the Resources section for monosaccharide supplements I recommend and visit our website, www.calciumlie.com, for updates and further information.

How much will it cost?

We'll be the first to admit, supplements and better quality foods can be pricey. You know your budget, but please do think of this program as an investment in a longer, healthier life, your most prized asset. Prioritize your budget with this in mind. You are worth it. Start with minerals and the whole-food C and maybe also iodine for reasons discussed in Chapters 5 and 6.

With some employers, you can set up a medical savings account that will allow you to pay for supplements in pretax dollars. That'll save you anywhere from 15 percent to 35 percent right off the top, depending on your tax bracket. You can also pay for your HTMA and consultation with your doctor from these funds without having to hassle with your insurance company.

Some insurance companies will pay for the HTMA test (they all should); some try to say it is "experimental or unproven." HOOEY! It is no longer experimental. Well actually, it never was. It has always accurately measured molecular content and gradually it has acquired more advanced applications due to advances in the technology. The same science is used on the Mars Rover and in every chemistry lab in the world, and called micro mass spectrophotometry. After over 1,000,000 tests, there is plenty of data to confirm the clinical observations as associated with various and specific patient symptoms, diagnosis and medical conditions and relate them to specific mineral deficiencies and imbalances. Most insurance companies will pay for a nutritional consultation. It's certainly worth filing a claim.

There is quite simply no test that will have a greater impact on your long term health. I tell all my patients that there is no such thing as a bad HTMA: "It's just good to have it and bad not to." Once you have the correct HTMA information, you can reliably make changes and supplement to truly improve your health.

Just be sure you are getting what you are paying for. You've been educated by this book and you now know when a nutritionist is feeding you a load of outdated malarkey. When you hear the no-salt, no-egg yolks, take-a-calcium-supplement type of recommendations, just run! Or tell them to read this text and do their homework. *You* are now smarter than your provider.

In my experience, no other test has the potential to change your health more significantly than a HTMA. Even most of my teenage patients change their diets after HTMA results, so get a reliable HTMA to find out what you have and don't have for sure and which minerals are out of balance. Take your minerals please, more than 3 grams per day. Supplement correctly and eat correctly according to your body's mineral needs.

When it comes to supplements, don't waste your money on so-called "supplements" that are actually drugs unless there is a specific need or indication. There may be times when those supplements are appropriate in a short-term situation, but like any prescription drug, their use should be as minimal as possible and for the shortest time possible. Use only whole-food products and go for the best. It will pay off in the long run in terms of your health and your pocketbook, too. See the Resources section or refer to our website www.calciumlie.com for my recommendations.

Budget and prioritize the supplements that you need to make a difference in your health. I find so many patients are already spending money on supplements that are not helping or are even harmful. I feel that it is part of my job as a physician to direct my patients to which supplements are good, and which ones will truly make a difference.

Finally, we urge you to do what you can now. Our health is essentially declining from the day we are born.

I often hear my patients say, "I am pretty healthy." This basically means in general that there is not a crisis or health problem recognized, yet. Why wait until you get one?

Start today doing at least one positive thing toward better health every day. You can be sure it is making a difference. Start with baby steps and you'll soon find yourself walking and finally, running. Little steps lead to bigger ones. In my experience, patients who do one thing will do two, then four, then eight. The achievement of improving healthfulness will eventually become a habit (remember, I call this "healthful congruence"). This will also rub off eventually on those you love, especially if they see you getting great results.

We admit the HTMA results and nutritional recommendations that accompany them can be a little overwhelming.

Don't let yourself be overwhelmed. Take the advice of the "old saws": How do you eat an elephant? Answer: One bite at a time.

Little changes or corrections in food-buying preferences based on your HTMA results, and thoughtful supplementation can bring about amazing results. It takes time, but most of my patients experience meaningful improvements in short order. This time factor for results may also depend on the level of deteriorization or deficiency one has achieved before applying this information. Start ASAP.

Care should be taken to consult with someone with experience in the application of the HTMA test recommendations, just like any other laboratory test. I tailor the diet and supplement recommendations for each patient and each result based on my specific knowledge of the patient's issues, knowledge of nutrition and biochemistry and my personal experience with various supplements and their effects on specific health issues.

Take charge of your health and take control of your life. Do what is important and do it well. You can make a difference in your health and regain vitality and energy in ways you never imagined were possible. My best patients often tell me, "I don't just feel like I'm getting healthier, I feel like I'm getting younger." This is the ultimate compliment and it is my continuous wish for all my patients and loved ones.

POINTS TO REMEMBER

✔ Get an HTMA. No other medical test has a greater chance to impact your health long term.

✔ Find a doctor who is conversant in interpreting and implementing HTMA results from the only reliable lab and the only one I recommend, TEI.

✔ Little changes based on HTMA results can produce big results over time. Improving one meal per day is a 33 percent improvement, two meals 66 percent, and three meals is a 99 percent improvement.

✔ Follow the six simple steps to better nutrition. Even if you can't do it at every meal, eat as well as you can, clean, organic vegetables and meats. Include a daily dose of monosaccharide-rich foods like maple syrup or sweet potatoes.

✔ Budget for supplements. You are worth it. Your health is your most important asset. At the very least, take the supplements that are the most important to and most likely to have the greatest impact on your health. They are, unfortunately, necessary today due to the nutritional deficiencies of our foods. It is nearly impossible today to eat to achieve optimal health without correct supplementation.

CHAPTER 10

Doctor to Doctor:
An Impassioned Plea

THROUGHOUT THIS BOOK, we've thrown out some—ahem—unconventional ideas about health, nutrition and the underlying causes of the diseases that are quite literally shortening our lives.

Everything in this book is based on solid, scientific evidence. There's nothing airy-fairy or mystical about it. Most of the premises in this book come from basic biochemistry, courses every doctor took in pre-med and medical school.

We'll be the first to tell you that many of these concepts are not well known or commonly accepted. Patients who take them to their doctors or nutritionists are likely to be summarily dismissed or even ridiculed. Your doctor might summarily veto your supplement regimen without any solid information or knowledge. Your nutritionist might tell you that your bones will crumble to dust if you don't take calcium supplements.

You've read this book. You *know* that your doctor and your nutritionist are operating on the voodoo wavelength and that we have presented you with solid science.

Doctors who espouse the commonsense solid scientific concepts presented in this book are likely to be ostracized by their colleagues. I know. I have been a victim of that sort of professional jealousy, jousting, personal attack, arrogance and intellectual dishonesty. This is still hard to accept.

Doctors generally choose what they want to believe like a religion, with little regard for each other and shamefully often with little regard for their patients. Protecting the status quo is paramount to them as is their income and avoiding lawsuits, not necessarily doing the right thing all the time. It is very difficult for them to see the impact of their exorbitant fees and the cost of the drugs they prescribe.

What is truly shocking is that two physicians with whom I had worked for years severely criticized *The Calcium Lie*, without ever having read it or checking a single reference. One physician didn't like the first edition's subtitle, *What Your Doctor Doesn't Know Might Kill You* because she "disagreed with the premise." The other based his criticism on only this chapter in the original text. He also disagreed with the reliability of HTMA, despite qualified expert opinions endorsing it and scientific, published, peer-reviewed technical and clinical material confirming its reliability. He chose instead to believe unscientific Internet websites (his sole source of references) of repeatedly plagiarized material and insurance company negative opinions. This is all true and so sadly indicative of the way most conventional doctors think today.

We can only offer this plea from the heart: **Please, doctors, read this book!**

Patients: By all means, read this chapter and read it closely. But we have really written this concluding chapter as an open letter to all doctors, as an impassioned plea for them to put aside their prejudices and their adherence to The Calcium Lie, The Vitamin Lie and a dozen or more other erroneous belief systems that are not scientifically based and begin to make a difference through good nutritional science and genuine caring.

If we as physicians are ever going to make a difference in the overall health of our patients, their surgical needs and outcomes, and their all-too-prevalent illnesses and diseases from pregnancy to old age, we must begin to address the significance of the nutritional lies made apparent through this work. Protecting the status quo should not be acceptable ever again when considering the dismal health statistics and outcomes we see in our societies today, not to mention exorbitant costs of the care required as a result and the incredible impact of the loss of wellness on our lives. Our illnesses are big business and there is quite literally no incentive to change this. Obamacare is not the answer. It does nothing to change disease statistics. It merely insures everyone pays more and creates more bureaucracy.

We urge you, with our blessings, to copy these pages of this book and give them to your doctor. Better yet, buy another copy and make it a gift.

Make your pleas for your physician to read these pages as impassioned as is our advocacy for you.

We know doctors are busy people, so we are making this chapter short and sweet to economize on valuable time; but doctors, we urge you to buy a copy of this book and read it in its entirety, challenge the assertions scientifically, check the compelling references—in short, do your homework. We think it will change your life, your practice and will be of great service to your patients. Who knows? Maybe it'll even help you improve your health and heal yourself. The basic truths in this book are irrefutable.

Dear Doctor,

Your patient has given you a copy of this chapter with our blessing and permission. We have given this chapter to public domain to try to get the truth out as quickly as possible about calcium and the other assertions of the text. We care that this vital information lands in your hands and that you give it your careful and thoughtful consideration.

We ask you to set aside your preconceived ideas or what you think you know is true and give these few pages your careful consideration.

We also ask you to spend ten minutes to read these pages all the way to the end. It is our fervent hope that they will change your professional life and profoundly affect the lives of your patients.

The majority of physicians practicing today are there because they made a choice to help people. I felt the same way. I was a bright-eyed, naïve, idealistic youngster who, at age 19 felt a special calling to the practice of medicine. Almost all of us had those altruistic motives when we entered medical school, but the way medicine is practiced today, those altruistic motives have been largely beaten out of us and more often greed has become a deciding factor.

With all our current taxes, liability and exorbitant overhead costs, practicing medicine is a lot like being a hamster on a wheel. You have to keep turning that wheel to stay ahead. Despite what most laypeople believe, a license to practice medicine is not a license to print money. In fact, there is absolutely no security in practicing medicine. It is basically a service occupation, with high overhead and high risk of legal liability, and very little security. Maybe I should call this The Big Bucks Doctor Lie.

Sure, some doctors are earning beaucoup bucks, but the average doctor is confronted with huge debts, big overheard expenses, enormous insurance premiums, no paid time off to rest, vacation and recuperate, and no paid health and retirement benefits.

And doctors are expected to be knowledgeable about everything medical, make snap decisions when we are exhausted and always be right. Yes, you can make a comfortable living, but you have to work hard for it and make sacrifices that most people would never consider.

If you're on that hamster wheel and feeling overwhelmed, go back to those days when you were a bright-eyed med student. It was your choice to become a physician. In my 31 years of practice, I've discovered something that borders on the mystical: Enough money keeps on coming as long as I work hard and make the right choices, even in the hard times, and yes, I have had them too. As long as I keep my sights on my mission to help my patients feel better and improve their health, my conscience is at peace.

I have been the victim of professional jealousy, anticompetitive behavior, vicious gossip and professional attacks by colleagues who apparently felt threatened by the success of my patients. The behavior I have witnessed and experienced firsthand in this regard merely for being a leader is quite simply despicable, to say the least.

In 1996, I was ready to throw in the towel, ready to stop competing with my colleagues, ready to give up on the insurance companies and quit medicine for good. I had no idea what I would do, but I was just sick of the way many in my chosen profession cannibalize each other over money, with totally uncompassionate and anticompetitive behavior, in the name of good medicine.

Sometimes, unfortunately, a physician or group of politically entrenched physicians will protect and cover up substandard practice behaviors arbitrarily and capriciously, in the name of peer review and financial gain.

In 1996, on one of my lowest days as a physician, a phone call came informing me that I had been chosen one of the "Best Doctors in America." What an honor! My spirits soared in a conflict of irony and my thoughts of leaving the profession were diminished. Maybe I could make a difference. Maybe I could take whatever criticism and heat my colleagues could dish out as long as someone recognized that I was actually doing what was right, what I *had originally* set out to do. I *was* helping my patients get better and it was being recognized nationally. I was somewhat re-energized!

The message of this book is basically a continuation of that excitement about the ability to create better care, to recognize many of the simple untruths that we practice and advocate incorrectly as a profession and once again, to try to reach physicians and call them back to the roots of their educations, far away from the influence of pharmaceutical companies and insurance regulations.

At about the same time, I realized that I had been developing an increased awareness and intellectual accountability for my pregnant patients who would come in and ask me about the nutritional supplements they were taking. They wanted to use various herbs and supplements, as well as prenatal "vitamins," and they wanted my recommendations about the best ones to take, and how much and which ones were safe.

These are the same questions we face as physicians every day concerning pharmaceuticals. I realized that I needed to practice the same due diligence in making these recommendations by educating myself about nutritional concepts and supplements with the same level of veracity that I would apply to any and all medication recommendations. Much of this information wasn't even in the books or taught when I was in medical school or, at least, not in the classes where I sat. I also needed to go back to my roots in basic science and biochemistry and apply what I did know to human nutrition and separate fact from fiction.

I'm pretty sure your experience in medical school was similar to mine: Out of thousands of classroom hours, we may have received four hours or less of instruction on human nutrition. Doctors are not "supposed" to have to know this "stuff." Yet this information is quite literally at the heart of how we treat our patients, no matter what our specialties. Virtually every disease process of the human body has a connection to nutritional imbalances, toxicities, shortfalls and deficiencies. Yet we spent so little time learning about nutrition in medical school that it is now time for us all to begin to re-educate ourselves. Our collective health and that of our patients demands it.

My award in 1996 not only re-energized me in my practice of medicine, I felt compelled to research other fields of medicine and nutritional products so I could provide my patients with the best possible care and guide them in what was safe, what works, what doesn't and what not to take. I started to learn more about herbs, supplements and other alternative therapies, including homeopathy.

Before you pooh-pooh homeopathy, think about it. The use of homeopathy or microscopic doses of various toxins or nontoxic substances with very specific effects to trigger an immune or physiological response works because these remedies are water-soluble and can be easily carried into the cells.

Think about your basic biochemistry and homeopathy will make sense to you. More importantly, it has been used for over two hundred years, has a scientific basis and, when used properly, it does no harm. If it works, great—use it. If it doesn't work some of the time, try something else. There is ample evidence-based medicine that it works. In my experience, homeopathic remedies work about 60 to 80 percent of the time in treating the symptoms. Remember, drugs don't always work either. This is simply an example. Homeopathy is not the answer. Like herbs, it merely treats the symptoms with less toxicity. We must recognize and treat the underlying problems to get our patients better and truly reverse them or best of all, to prevent disease from developing in the first place.

We as physicians need to be accountable for all the practices of our field, all the science, not just that which we believe. The future of our civilization is truly at stake. I am continually challenged by what I do not know. To fail to re-examine and question the science of "what you believe is true" is practicing a religion, not a science. We have to doubt that which we think we know to advance our knowledge. Each answer should raise new and more profound questions.

Part of my examination based on my patients' requests for more natural ways to approach pregnancy and childbirth showed me that there was an impressive amount of medical knowledge regarding the use of herbs in medicine that are often the basis for our drugs. They have various effects, good and bad, some even stimulate immune responses, but like homeopathy and drugs, herbs as whole-foods largely treat symptoms but with less toxicity. Like homeopathy, herbs are not *the* answer, but they can be helpful when beneficial and safe.

Eventually, I realized The Calcium Lie and its links to mineral deficiencies, excesses, imbalances and disease.

In a nutshell, The Calcium Lie says that bones are not made of calcium alone, but of at least 12 minerals, including calcium. Expecting to keep bones strong by giving someone calcium supplements is like expecting that you can make a loaf of bread from yeast alone. It simply won't work. In the case of the use of, or recommendation for, calcium supplements, this lie can do great harm as crystallized excess calcium concretions make their way into arteries and joints; this forces the adrenals to compensate for the calcium excess to their own detriment. This problem leads to a continuous decline in sodium and potassium from the body, changes in cell membrane physiology and electrical potential, and causes the brain to shrink and become demented. More and more studies have validated the dangers of excess intracellular calcium since the publication of the first edition of this book in 2008.

We're not going to rehash this entire book here, but we're going to repeat The Calcium Cascade from Chapter 2, since you may have received these copied pages from a patient (with our blessings) and you may not yet have access to the entire book. The chart may help trigger some recollections for you of how and why the biochemical process we describe in this book is perfectly logical, based on the biochemistry classes you took in medical school.

It leads to a simple conclusion: Almost everyone needs trace minerals, not just calcium, because we simply cannot get all nutrients we need from food grown in our minerally depleted soils, picked before ripeness, especially in view of our society's propensity for nutritionally void foods. And most importantly: Calcium hardens concrete, not bones. Excess calcium can do severe damage to the human organism, especially the brain, arteries and other soft tissue.

The Calcium Cascade

Excess calcium in the human body begins a cascade of negative effects that have enormous adverse consequences to our health. This process cannot be diagnosed with standard blood tests. It requires a reliable, competent lab to conduct a tissue mineral analysis on a correctly collected hair sample you provide. I recommend Trace Elements Inc., the only lab with the correct ratios and databases. You can find information about them in the Resources section and through my website, www.calciumlie.com.

If you have excess or relative calcium excess in your body

THAT LEADS TO

Calcium seeking and needing more magnesium to try to keep your body's calcium and magnesium in balance

THAT LEADS TO

A relative magnesium deficiency in proportion to calcium that leads to increased muscle tension and nerve endings firing erratically and other "electrical" malfunctions in your body;

AND

In its need for more magnesium, your body has to suppress adrenal function in order to retain more magnesium to compensate for the high calcium; This adrenal suppression causes a continuous loss of sodium and potassium in your urine as well as immune compromise from the adrenal suppression.

THIS LEADS TO

A continual depletion of the sodium and potassium that are stored inside the trillions of cells in your body;

THAT LEADS TO

A loss of the sodium and chloride you need to produce the stomach acid you need to digest protein;

AND

This increases the incidences of heartburn and other digestive disorders, and the use of prescription drugs that have further destructive effects and impede digestion;

AND

Your body gradually loses its ability to digest protein and absorb the essential amino acids that are the building blocks of protein and neurotransmitters.

ALSO

The sodium depletion leads to a failure of membrane electrical potential and ion exchanges necessary for cellular function, the mechanism by which our bodies get essential amino acids and glucose into all our cells, except fat cells, which keep absorbing glucose without sodium while the rest of our bodies' cells are starving.

FURTHERMORE

Intracellular potassium levels decline dramatically and this leads to increasing degrees of thyroid hormone resistance (type 2 hypothyroidism), with all the symptoms of hypothyroidism and slowed metabolism with what are thought to be normal blood tests. Correct diagnosis requires blood tests, HTMA, basal body temperatures and total and reverse T3 ratio.

SO

All cells (except fat cells) become starved for glucose and amino acids,

RESULTING IN

Increased cravings for glucose and increased food intake.
This loss of minerals also leads to more food cravings

AND

Intracellular deficiencies of sodium, potassium and essential amino acids, and more cravings.

THE END RESULT IS

Multiple metabolic malfunctions, including obesity, heart disease, type 2 hypothyroidism, type 2 diabetes, anxiety, migraines, depression, dementia, hypertension
and the list goes on and on!

When I re-examined my biochemistry and physiology thinking, I remembered the simple truth of this basic physiology, which I call the Calcium Cascade. It triggered insatiable curiosity in me. I began to quickly build my knowledge about nutrition and supplements, something I am somewhat ashamed to confess I had pooh-poohed to my patients in the past, just like so many other physicians. I began to discover what worked and what didn't in nutrition and supplements. I saw the results in my patients and myself and I was encouraged to persist.

I had to struggle to overcome the brainwashing I had received on The Calcium Lie. The simple question recurring in my head was,

"Why had such an error in basic scientific truth and teaching become so entrenched in medical thinking and practice?"

I dug deeper and I found out about hair tissue mineral analysis (HTMA) application, about how scientifically reliable it actually is and how validated laboratory certified testing methods could provide me with a wealth of information about a patient's medical conditions. The HTMA also provides diagnostic clues and helps me to address them nutritionally, often reversing the problems.

I carefully examined the websites with plagiarized misinformation and out-of-date and misleading science pooh-poohing the reliability of HTMA. I also sought out the current knowledge on HTMA science. I did my scientific homework on the technology of micro-mass spectrophotometry, its applications, its reliability and its usefulness in practicing medicine. This is the same technology that is now being applied to bacteriology and has revolutionized microbiology in the last 10 years, although it is still not widely applied. With this technology, bacteria can now be identified in about 45 seconds accurately. At least 7,000 so far have been clearly "fingerprinted." This advance is huge, thanks to the same technology used in HTMA.

I began to look at the effectiveness of each treatment. Even more importantly, I searched for treatments for conditions that often had no good options and often went unaddressed or for which there were only drugs to treat symptoms. If one treatment wasn't working, I searched for alternatives and networked with other like-minded professionals to find out if they had any answers and to learn from their experiences and absorb their opinions. I continue to do so.

I also became acutely aware that I was required to label patients with their afflictions. Someone with diabetes became a diabetic and was labeled accordingly. That's how we are trained. That's how we are paid. But as I began to change my way of thinking, I realized that there are no diseases we are "supposed" to have and that almost all of these labels are related to nutritional deficiencies and imbalances which, when corrected, cause the illness(es) to remit or resolve. This increased awareness opened a whole new way of thinking for me, a whole new approach to my patients, and has helped them immeasurably. That's so much more like the ideals that I had originally set out to practice as a physician.

As a little aside, I'll tell you that as soon as I began to change my way of thinking about diabetes and started treating the nutritional and mineral deficiencies and imbalances in patients with type 2 diabetes and insulin resistance, I began to achieve phenomenal success.

Over the past 16 years, my treatment plan has kept blood sugars normal in more than 100 patients with diagnosed type 2 diabetes without pharmaceuticals, and has done so effectively over long periods of time. This program is effective for virtually everyone with insulin resistance and every overweight person. If caught and treated early in the course of the disease, I have found that insulin resistance is nearly always reversible. Based on my experience, if the diagnosis of severe insulin resistance as type 2 diabetes has taken place in the past two years, the disease is nearly always reversible. If the diagnosis is more than two and less than five years old, type 2 diabetes is still sometimes reversible. If the diagnosis has been made more than five years in the past, my treatment plan may not be able to reverse the disease, but it can result in improved blood sugar control.

Joe R was one of these patients with recent onset type 2 diabetes. His fasting blood sugars were from 150 to 250 and postprandial sugars from 250 to 400. With immediate and correct supplementation, within two weeks all his blood sugars were normal and, with continued diet and supplement regimens, have remained so for more than 16 years.

For Joe and these other patients, the key was correct supplementation with the appropriate supplements to reduce insulin resistance, not just prescribing drugs to sensitize the patient's body to the overproduction of insulin, which increases fat cell glucose absorption. That means treating and reversing the underlying problem with the correct supplements, not drugs. Chromium picolinate doesn't work, at least not very well, but chromium polynicotinate (ChromeMate™) does.

I don't expect the dairy and pharmaceutical industries and the supplement companies will like this book much, since it is challenging you to think and move away from the erroneous belief systems that they have so carefully nurtured.

No doubt, I will be personally attacked for my conviction and new direction in patient care. It's OK. I have pretty broad shoulders and thick skin and lots of faith. I have always been a leader. Doing the right thing for the right reasons has always been important to me. To the doctors who have criticized me for being a leader, please understand I have been right before about laparoscopy, Curaderm and now The Calcium Lie. This is just plain fact. I made simple observations and I am reporting them again, with even more evidence and more conviction in this edition than what I documented in the first edition of this book in 2008.

We have struggled in the writing of this book to put these concepts into simple terms that the average reader can comprehend. If we have oversimplified, we will take responsibility for that. Of course, biochemistry is very complex. There is no doubt that physicians are among the most educated and intelligent people in the world, and we know that they can take these simplified concepts and apply what they learned in medical school to acknowledge these truths.

I take intellectual honesty with great seriousness. I cannot have a knee-jerk reaction to a patient's question about a supplement, medication, surgery or any type of treatment. That knee-jerk reaction would be based on what I *think* I know and not necessarily on science. I continually take myself back to my roots in med school biochemistry and ferret out the answers based on science, not advertising or drug rep dinners or just "knowing" or believing something.

Before this goes too far, I want to say I don't consider supplements to be a panacea. In fact, many supplements are actually drugs, and as such can be harmful. This is the subject of Chapter 7 of this book, The Vitamin Lie, which says that we've been duped into believing that a single component of an extraordinarily complex molecule that comprises a vitamin is the vitamin itself. Case in point: Vitamin C is *not* ascorbic acid, although almost all vitamin C supplements sold on the market today are just that, ascorbic acid, not vitamin C. Unless someone takes in the whole vitamin C molecule harvested from 100 percent whole-foods, vine ripened and grown in mineral-rich soils, your patients won't be getting the benefits of this remarkable life-giving vitamin and will suffer the consequences.

This is my plea to you: Remember your roots. Remember who you are and how you were trained. Remember your early education, especially your biochemistry, however painful this may be.

Put aside belief systems about medicine and open your mind to what some may think are "new" ways of thinking, but which are actually just basic, solid science.

I remember a fairly pompous medical school professor in my early days of medical school who told us that only 20 percent of everything that we were going to be taught was true. The only problem was that they didn't know which part was the 20 percent that was true—and neither did we. Maybe that one caveat contained more wisdom than I realized at the time.

Erase The Calcium Lie from your mind. Press the delete key in your brain. You *know* that bones are not made of calcium and you know that osteoporosis is the loss of minerals from the bones, not just the loss of calcium. Then treat your patients accordingly. See that they get a complete complement of trace minerals based on basic scientific evidence, and even better, based on hair tissue mineral analysis results from a reputable laboratory.

After all, isn't bone mineral density just another way of clinically measuring tissue mineral levels—in this case, in bone? Think about it. Bone density is just a general measurement of the total mineral content of the bone; the HTMA gives us the specific levels of all the most important minerals and their balance for the entire body. I have found HTMA mineral levels correlate quite closely with osteopenia and osteoporosis, with lots more useful information.

The only lab I trust completely to accurately measure whole body tissue mineral levels is Trace Elements, Inc. (www.traceelements.com or by phone at 800-824-2314 or through my website at www.calciumlie.com).

Dr. David Watts, founder of Trace Elements, Inc., has developed a database of more than 1,000,000 hair tissue samples from which he has extrapolated highly accurate predictions of disease risk based upon the basic science of known relationships of mineral deficiencies, excesses, imbalances and toxic ratios to known clinical disease and medical science. Find out your patients' mineral deficiencies and imbalances, and you'll be able to begin treating them medically and nutritionally with reliable, reproducible and gratifying success.

When you rearrange your thinking process, you can treat your patients as you did when you were a bright-eyed med student. Begin to question what you *think* you know.

You can re-energize your practice of medicine, care a little more about your patients and actually help them get better, rather than just treating their symptoms, as the pharmaceutical industry would encourage you to do.

Not everything that comes from the drug companies or supplement companies is good—nor is it all bad. We need to educate ourselves to discern what is good and what is not and whenever possible, treat the underlying issue. This is our sworn responsibility as physicians.

We as physicians have great power to help or to hurt. It is our choice how we will treat our patients and how we will, ultimately, make a difference in their lives, our lives and the world. If you use this information with honesty, honor and integrity, you'll attract more patients than you can imagine. My medical practice has morphed into a practice that is about 90 percent nutritionally based, with many men and children joining my women patients.

This book is a gift to you. Take and use this information with our blessings for you and your patients.

—From *The Calcium Lie* by Robert Thompson, M.D.,
and Kathleen Barnes (Take Charge Books, 2013)
Website: www.calciumlie.com

Resources

Since we're forging new territory here, the resources we can offer are a process. I would potentially endorse any product that provides me with an independent Certificate of Analysis (COA) that confirms by third party that the vitamin or the supplement is the pure bioidentical molecule as the whole-food. This should be our standard. We hope that in the coming months and years, we'll be able to flesh out this list and offer you more resources for everything you need to combat The Calcium Lie and find your way back to health. The best resource to date is probably AuroraHealthandNutrition .com, where I am continuously updating my recommendations. These are the products I personally have experience with that work.

The best way for you to keep up with the latest information is to visit www.calciumlie.com often and subscribe to our newsletter at www.calcium-lie.com/newsletter.

I know there are many other good products on the market. But we need to know: Are they really necessary? Are they going to make a difference? Are the basic metabolic needs being satisfied? Are they good but not needed? Or are they potentially harmful, as in "vitamin" C (as ascorbic acid), the substitute, and the potentially harmful real vitamin C–depleting chemical substance called ascorbic acid.

I have included in this list the products that I know and trust through my years of clinical practice. I continually re-evaluate these products and compare them to new emerging products. These products have consistently performed well in my patients when taken correctly. And they are, to the best of my knowledge, 100 percent whole-food bioidentical molecules in every case.

WEBSITES

My websites: www.calciumlie.com
www.aurorahealthandnutrition.com
www.drt-obgyn.com

WHERE TO FIND A GOOD DOCTOR

First, check our website, www.calciumlie.com. We hope to post an ever-growing list of physicians who are equipped to help you.

The American College for Advancement in Medicine, an association of integrative health practitioners: www.acam.org, phone: 949-309-3520.

The American Academy of Anti-Aging Medicine (A4M), has doctors worldwide who are dedicated to preventive health. They also have a fellowship program for training and certifying antiaging practicing physicians: www.worldhealth.net, phone: 773-528-1000.

Insulin Potentiation Therapy website: While this website is dedicated to a specific form of complementary or alternative cancer treatment, the medical doctors who administer this treatment are open-minded and progressive and likely to be able to help you to rebalance your minerals: www.iptforcancer.com.

Robert Thompson, M.D. Call the office at 907-260-6914 to schedule a nutritional consultation or to obtain an HTMA test

HAIR TISSUE MINERAL ANALYSIS (HTMA) TESTS

Trace Elements, Inc., is reliable, trustworthy and accurate. Their database is the largest in the world. HTMA kits can be ordered through:
www.calciumlie.com
www.aurorahealthandnutrition.com
Robert Thompson, M.D., 907-260-6914

NATURAL SEA SALT

These are the best brands of natural and unrefined sea salt:

Celtic sea salt: www.celticseasalt.com

Redmond sea salt: www.realsalt.com

(Available in supermarkets and health food stores, Celtic sea salt is available through www.aurorahealthandnutrition.com.)

Infused sea salts are delightful for cooking, such as Alderwood Smoked Sea Salt on fish or chicken, Hickory Smoked Sea Salt on meat or game, Habanero Sea Salt on everything, Chipolte Sea Salt on barbecue, Merlot Sea Salt on steak. Also there are many other flavors such as Black Truffle, French Gray, and on and on. If you know you need it, enjoy the delights in flavor.

Fortisalt Spray (is magnificent on everything, especially salads, adds balanced trace minerals to your food and is sodium neutral ($1/3$ of normal, so not bitter).

VITAMIX

A Vitamix machine is much more than a blender. It can process fruits, vegetables, even grains so that you can easily assimilate the maximum nutrients available in your food. Nutrient absorption is related to particle size, so the specific degree of blending power of this machine is that which is most likely to produce the smallest particles of food while leaving in the all-important fiber: www.vitamix.com.

SUPPLEMENTS

www.aurorahealthandnutrition.com

www.calciumlie.com

www.drt-obgyn.com

www.calciumlie2.com

For other products and companies I recommend or for specific information regarding their use in my practice, please refer to www.aurorahealthandnutrition .com:

A.C. Grace Company: www.acgrace.com

Unique E

AlgaeCal: www.algaecal.com
AlgaeCal(plant calcium plus minerals,
   from *Algas Calcareas*)

Allergy Research Group:
  www.allergyresearchgroup.com
Oregano Oil
Organic Germanium

Bob's Red Mill Natural Foods:
  www.bobsredmill.com
Stabilized Rice Bran

Body Health: www.bodyhealth.com
Metal Free (special order).

Chi Enterprises: www.chi-health.com
Myomin
Prostate Chi

Wayne Garland:
  www.masterformulas.net
Diabetic Glucose Control Formula
Imperial Qi
Ocean Gold (shark liver oil)
Topical Shark Liver Oil

Innate Response:
www.innateresponse.com
B-complex (100 percent whole-food)
C-complex (100 percent whole-food)
Pre/Postnatals (100 percent whole-food)

Klearsen Corporation Peaceful Mountain:
www.peacefulmountain.com
Eczema Relief Cream
Cold Sore Remedy

Life Extension: www.lef.org
Cognitex (increased memory possible)
Cinsulin
Weight Control Formula

Mannatech: us.mannatech.com
(control #456515 to order)
Ambrotose Powder (plain)
Emprisone Cream

Natural Partners:
www.naturalpartners.com
7 keto-DHEA 25 mg and 50 mg
(special order)
Eurocel (special order, for use in
Hepatitis C)
Germanium
Rhyzinate
Vitex

Quincy Bioscience:
www.quincybioscience.com
Prevagen 40 mg

ProThera: www.protherainc.com
"Pure Encapsulations"
Alpha Lipoic Acid 600 mg tabs
ChromeMate 600 mcg tabs 180
capsules
DHEA 10 mg, 25 mg, and 50 mg caps
Eciosamax (ultrapure omega-3)
gel caps

Glucosamine 750 mg capsules
5-HTP 50 mg caps
Indole Forte 400 mg caps
Iodine 12.5 mg capsules (Iodide
and Iodine)
MSM 750 mg caps
Vitamin D3, 1000 IU capsules

Researched Nutritionals:
www.researchednutritionals.com
CO-Q10
Inflamaquel
NT Factor Energy
Transfer Factor Multi-Immune
ATP Mitochondrial Fuel
Transfer Factor Energy
Sanesco
Adaptagen
Contegra
Lentra
Methyl Max
Prolent
Somni TR
Tranquelent
Corvalen
D-Ribose

True Botanica:
www.truebotanica.com
Berberine 500 mg

The Grain Society: (available retail
in various locations, including
online)
Celtic Sea Salt
Thera Biotic Probiotics
Lactobacillus (25 billion live
multispecies)

Thorne Research: www.thorne.com
L-Tyrosine
Perfusia (sustained release
L-arginine)

Trace Mineral Research: www.traceminerals.com

Trace Minerals ("blue bottle"-standard formula, correct for everyone, but not corrective for those with low potassium, liquid and caplet form)

Electrolyte formula ("red label"-the same minerals, in the same balance, but with extra potassium).

Only the product with my name on it is formulated correctly, liquid or caplet form, corrective for those with low intracellular potassium and mineral deficiency).

Vitamin Only (created for me by Innate Response, this is the first 100 percent whole-food multivitamin without added minerals, therefore the correct multi-formula of whole-food vitamins for every man, woman, and child that can swallow caplets safely regardless of body mineral content).

Available through my website: www.aurorahealthandnutrition.com

SPECIFIC NUTRIENTS

Trace Minerals Ionic Sea Salt–Derived Minerals:
I like the ionic minerals produced by a company called Trace Minerals Research because I know they are safe, absorbable and effective. I admit they are a bit difficult to find, so I am offering them through my website. There are a couple of other products that are of good quality, so I'm including them here. You can also get them through my website and the other websites listed.

www.aurorahealthandnutrition.com

www.mineralresourcesint.com

www.traceminerals.com

www.originalquinton.com

Whole-food vitamin C
Innate vitamin C (100 percent whole-food vitamin C). This product is only sold through doctors' offices. You can get it at my website:www.aurorahealthand nutrition.com

Monosaccharides
Ambrotose—Manantech
Control number: #456515
www.aloewholesale.com (Improve U.S.A., Inc.)
www.aurorahealthandnutrition.com
This is the only monosaccharide product I have been able to find. If anyone knows of other products, please let us know through our website, www.calciumlie.com.

Maple Syrup (food source of monosaccharides):
Look for products that are 100 percent pure maple syrup, including:
www.dennisfarmsmaple.com
www.maplesource.com

Whole-Food Vitamins (formulated to my specifications):
www.aurorahealthandnutritionl.com

To treat specific conditions: all available at www.aurorahealthandnutrition.com

REFLUX AND GERD

Rhyzonate

HYPERTENSION

Profusia (sustained-release L-arginine)
Ocean Gold (shark liver oil)

TYPE 2 DIABETES

ChromeMate, Diabetic Glucose Control Formula

ESSENTIAL FATTY ACID DEFICIENCIES

Eciosamax (ultrapure omega-3)
Ocean Gold (shark liver oil)

OTHER PRODUCTS

Water Filters:
Aquasana: www.aquasana.com
Jonathan Beauty Water Filtration:
www.jonathanproduct.com/home.html

Alkalinizing Water Filters:
AKAI
KYK Genesis
High Tech Health
Kaegan
www.aurorahealthandnutrition.com

References

Note to Readers

While there is good scientific research to back the theories presented in this book, all of the principles of The Calcium Lie, the effects of mineral deficiencies, insufficiencies and excesses, are found in basic biochemistry. Any college biochemistry textbook will confirm every word in this book, extrapolated logically. This is why I am so dismayed that physicians who have studied these basic scientific truths in depth seem to choose to "forget" the basic science that they learned in medical school and buy into the medical myths presented in *The Calcium Lie 2*. Here are references that will help.

BOOKS

Anderson, F., *Nature's Answer—Replenish The Earth*, Replenishing Press, Bear River, Utah, 84301, 2001.

Audhya, Tapan, *Role of B Vitamins in Biologic Methylation*, Health Diagnostics and Research Institute (Vitamin Diagnostics, Inc.).

Barnes, Kathleen, *10 Best Ways to Manage Stress*, Take Charge Books, 2013.

The Brain Health Guide, by Quincy Bioscience 2012.

Brownstein, David, *Iodine, Why You Need It, Why You Can't Live Without It*, Medical Alternatives Press, 2009.

Brownstein, David, *Salt Your Way to Health*, Medical Alternatives Press, 2006.

Campbell, Colin and Thomas, Colin, *The China Study*, Benbella Books, 2006.

DeCava, M. L., *The Real Truth About Vitamins and Antioxidants*, A. Printery, 1997.

Gaby, Alan R. and Wright, Jonathan V., *Nutritional Therapy in Medical Practice, Reference Manual and Study Guide*, Nutrition Seminars, 2011.

Kabara, Jon J., *Fats Are Good for You and Other Secrets*, North Atlantic Books, 2008.

Lee, John, *What Your Doctor May Not Tell You About Menopause*, Warner Books 1996.

Marx, David, *Wack a Mole*, By Your Side Studios, Aug., 2009.

Mc Daniel, A. B., *The New Enocrinology: New Applications of Current Research for Integrative Solutions*, Nov., 2011.

Russell, M. R., *What the Bible Says About Healthy Living*, Regal Books, 2001.

Sapolsky, R., *Why Zebras Don't Get Ulcers*, Holt Paperbacks, Aug., 2004.

Starr, M. M., *Hypothyroidism, Type 2, The Epidemic*, New Voice Publication, 2005.

Wallach, Joel and Lan, Ma, *Rare Earths, Forbidden Cures*, Wellness Publications, 1994.

Watts, David L., *Trace Elements and Other Essential Nutrients*, Writer's B-L-O-C-K, 2006.

Wright, Jonathan and Lenard, Lane, *Why Stomach Acid is Good for You*, M. Evans and Co., 2001.

Wright, Johnathan V. and Morgenthaler, John, *Natural Hormone Replacement*, Smart Publications, 1997.

Young, Robert O. and Young, Shelly Redford, *The pH Miracle, Balance Your Diet, Reclaim Your Health*, Grand Central Life and Style, 2010.

ARTICLES

Chapter 1:

Bolland, M.J., "Effect of calcium supplements on risk of myocardial infarction and cardiovascular events: a meta-analysis," *British Medical Journal*, 2010:341.c3691.

Bolland M.J., Barber P.A., et al. Vascular events in healthy older women receiving calcium supplementation: randomised controlled trial. *BMJ*. 2008 Feb 2;336(7638):262–6. doi: 10.1136/bmj.39440.525752.BE. Epub 2008 Jan 15.

Buchberger, W., Effects of sodium bromine on the biosynthesis of thyroid hormones and brominated/iodinated thyronines," *J. Trace Elem. Elec. Health Dis.*, Vol. 4. 1990 pp. 25–30.

Gallagher, C., "Hypercalcuria and stone risk with calcium and vitamin D supplementation," 94th Endocrine Society Annual Meeting, June 2012.

"Heart disease and calcium and vitamin D supplementation," *Heart*, May 24, 2012.

Horowitz, B., "Brominism from excessive cola consumption," *Clinical Toxicology*, 35 (3), 315–320, 1997.

Khachaturian, Z.S. "Hypothesis on the regulation of cytosol calcium concentration and the aging brain," *Neurobiology of Aging*, 8(4), 345–346, 1987.

Levin, M., "Bromine psychosis: four varieties," *Am. J. Psych.* 104:798–804, 1948.

Ling, G. N., "Truth in basic biomedical science will set future mankind free," *Physiol Chem Phys and Med*, NMR, (2011) 41:19–48.

Pavalka, S., "Effect of high bromine levels in the organism on the biological half-life of iodine in the rat. *Biol. Trace elem.* Res. 2001, Summer;82(1–3):133.

Raus, A.G., "Pharmacokinetics of bromine ion-an overview" *Chem. Toxic.*, Vol. 21, No. 1., 379, 1983.

Reid, Ian, "Calcium Supplements May Increase the Risk of Heart Disease," *British Medical Journal*, January 16, 2001.

Ried, I.R., "Does Calcium supplementation increase cardiovascular risk?" *Clinical Endocrinology*, Vol. 73, Issue 6, December 2010, pages 689–695.

Soremark, R., "Excretion of bromine ions by human urine," *Acta. Physiol. Scand.*, 50;306., 1960.

WHO and CIA Health Statistics, 2012.

Wilcox, D.C., et al., "gender gap in health span and life expectancy in okinawa: health behaviors," *Asian Journal of Gerontology and Geriatrics*, 2012; 7:49–58.

Chapter 2:

Golumb BA, Evans MA et al. Effects of statins on energy and fatigue with exertion: results from a randomized controlled trial. *Arch Intern Med.* 2012 Aug 13;172(15):1180-2. doi: 10.1001/archinternmed.2012.2171.

Healy, M., *Los Angeles Times*, Aug 24, 2011, IMS Health Source, 355 million statin prescriptions.

Kalantar-Zadeh K, Block G et al. Reverse epidemiology of conventional cardiovascular risk factors in patients with chronic heart failure. *J Am Coll Cardiol.* 2004 Apr 21;43(8):1439-44.

Lasardis, A.N., Sofos, A.B., "Calcium diet supplementation increases urinary sodium excretion in essential hypertension," *Nephron* 1987;45:250.

Leonhauser, M., "Managed-care coverage still at the heart of cardiovascular market," PM360online.com, FebRuary, 2012: pages 30–31.

Lundell, Dwight, Interview, "The true cause of heart disease," www.totalhealthbreakthroughs.com.

McLean, D.S., Ravid, S., et al. Effect of statin dose on incidence of atrial fibrillation: data form the Pravastatin or Atorvastatin Evaluation and Infection Therapy-Thrombolysis in Miycardial Infarction 22 (PROVE IT-TIMI 22) and Aggrastat to Zocor (A to Z) trials. *American Heart Journal* 2008 Feb;155(2):298–302.

Mohaupt, M.G., et al., *Canadian Medical Association Journal*, 181(1–2) E11–E18, Jul 2009.

Petursson, H, Sigardsson JA et al. Is the use of cholesterol in mortality risk algorithms in clinical guidelines valid? Ten years prospective data from the Norwegian HUNT 2 study. *J Eval Clin Pract.* 2012 Aug;18(4):927-8. doi: 10.1111/j.1365-2753.2012.01863.x.

Rea, T.D., et al., "Statin use and the risk of incident dementia: The cardiovascular health study," *Arch Neurol.* 62, 2005.

Ruperez, M., Lorenzo O et al. Connective Tissue growth factor is a mediator of angiotensin II-induced fibrosis. *Circulation* 2003 Sep 23;108(12):1499-505.

Saremi A, Bahn G., et al. Progression of vascular calcification is increased with statin use in the Veterans Affairs Diabetes Trial (VADT). *Diabetes Care.* 2012 Nov;35(11):2390-2. doi: 10.2337/dc12-0464. Epub 2012 Aug 8.

Sneff, S., "How statins really work, explains why they don't really work," ACAM, November 2012.

Tilvis, R.S., et al., *Annals of Medicine*, 2011.

Sifferlin, A., "Breaking down GlaxoSmithKline Billion-Dollar Wrongdoing," *Time, Health and Family*, July 5, 2012.

Yeboah, J, McClelland RL et al. Comparison of novel risk markers for improvement in cardiovascular risk assessment in intermediate-risk individuals. *JAMA.* 2012 Aug 22;308(8):788-95. doi: 10.1001/jama.2012.9624.

Chapter 3:

Bolland M.J., Barber P.A., et al. Vascular events in healthy older women receiving calcium supplementation: randomized controlled trial. *British Medical Journal* 2008 Feb. 2;336 (7638):262–6.

Kim, S.Y., et al., "Biosphosphonates and risk of atrial fibrillation: A meta-analysis," *Arthritis Research and Therapy*, 2010; 12(1):R30.

Seely, S. Is calcium excess in western diet a major cause of arterial disease? *International Journal of Cardiology* 1992 May;35(2):281–3.

Seely, S. Possible connection between milk and coronary heart disease:" The calcium hypothesis. *Medical Hypotheses* 2000 May;54(5):701–3.

Seely, S. The connection between lactose and coronary artery disease. *International Journal of Cardiology* 1994 Oct;48(2):199–207.

Seely, E.W., Graves, S.W. Calcium homoestasis in normotensive and hypertensive pregnancy. *Comprehensive Therapy* 1993;19(3):124–8.

Seely, S. Is calcium excess in western diet a major cause of arterial disease? *International Journal of Cardiology* 1991 Nov;33(2): 191–8.

Seely, S. On arterial calcification. *International Journal of Cardiology* 1997 Sep 19;61(2):105–8.

Chapter 4:

Audhya, T., "Role of B vitamins in biological methylation," Health Diagnostics and Research Institute.

Gilson, G., "Transmethylation: Often overlooked; critically important," ACAM Conference, Nov., 2007.

Grinwald, P., "Sodium pump failure in hypoxia and reoxygenation," *Journal of Molecular and Cellular Cardiology*, Dec., 1992; 24(12):1393–1398.

Ling, G. N., "Truth in basic biomedical science will set future mankind free," *Physiol Chem Phys and Med*, NMR, (2011) 41:19–48.

Seely S. The connection between milk and mortality from coronary heart disease, *Journal of Epidemiology and Community Health* 2002 DFec;56(12);958.

Chapter 5:

Asvold, B.O., et al., "The association between thyroid stimulating hormone (TSH) within the reference range and serum lipid concentrations in a population based study," The Hunt Study, *European Journal of Endocrinology*, 2007 Feb.; 156(2): 181–186.

Bernal, J., "Thyroid hormones and brain development," *Vitamins and Hormones*, 2005; 71:95–122.

Bowthorpe, J. A. *Stop the Thyroid Madness*, 2nd edition, Laughing Grape Publishing, 2012.

Carmen, M.T., et al. "Relationship of subclinical thyroid disease to the incidence of gestational diabetes," *Obstetrics and Gynecology*, Vol. 119(5), May 2012.

Cerilto, A., et al., "Free triiodothyronine: a novel predictor of postoperative atrial fibrilation," *European Journal of Cardiothoracic Surgery*, 2003; 24(4):487–492.

Danzi, S., et al., "Thyroid hormone treatment to mend a broken heart," *Jorunal of Clinical Endocrinology and Metabolism*, 2008, Apr.; 93(4):1172–1174.

Danzi, S., et al, "Thyroid hormone and the cardiovascular system," *Minerva Endocrinology*, 2004; 29(3):139–150.

Danzi, S., et al., "Parenteral uses of T3 in the treatment of human disease," Clinical Cornerstone, 2005; 7(2):59–115.

Dolidze, N.M., Kezeli, D.D.F., et al. "Changes in intra- and extracellular Ca2+ concentration and prostaglandin E2 synthesis in osteoblasts of the femoral bone in experimental hyper- and hypothyroidism," *Bulletin of Experimental Biology and Medicine* 2007 Jul;144(1):17–20.

Forti, P., et al., "Serum thyroid stimulating hormone as a predictor of cognitive impairment in an elderly cohort," *Gerontology*. 2011.

Friberg, L., et al., "Association between increased levels of reverse triiodothyronine (RT3) and mortality after acute myocardial infarction," *American Journal of Medicine*, 2001; 111(9): 699–703.

Gerdes, A., et al., "Thyroid replacement therapy and heart failure," *Circulation*, 2010; 122:385–393.

Grinwald P., "Sodium pump failure in hypoxia and reoxygenation," *Journal of Molecular and Cellular Cardiology*, 1992 Dec;24(12):1393–8.

Hak, A., et al., "Subclinical hypothyroidism is an independent risk factor for atherosclerosis and myocardial infarction in elderly women: The Rottendam Study," *Annals of Internal Medicine*, 2000; 132(4):270–278.

Hertoghe, T., "Lab tests, how to interpret them," Bioidentical Hormone Replacement Symposium, Las Vegas, Feb. 2013. Pg 435–436.

Holtorf, K., "Reverse T3 is the best measurement of thyroid tissue levels," *Journal of Clinical Endocrinology and Metabolism*, Vol. 90, 200

Iervasi G., et al., "Low T3 syndrome, a strong prognostic predictor of death in patients with heart disease," *Circulation*, 2003; 107:708.

Lambrubiydaki, I., et al., "High normal TSH in association with arterial stiffness in healthy postmenopausal women," *Journal of Hypertension*, 2012; 30(3):592–599.

Montero-Pedrazuela, A., et al., "Modulation of adult hippocampal neurogenesis by thyroid hormones: implications in depressive-like behavior," *Molecular Psychiatry*, 2006; 11:361–371.

Seely S., The connection between milk and mortality from coronary heart disease. *Journal of Epidemiology and Community Health* 2002 DFec;56(12);958.

Shimoyama, N., et al., "Serum thyroid hormone levels correlate with cardiac function and ventricualar tachyarythmia in patients with chronic heart failure," *Journal of Cardiology*, 1993: 23(2):205–213.

Wilson, E. D., *Wilson's Temperature Syndrome—A Reversible Low Temperature Problem*, Cornerstone Publishing, 1992.

Zulewski, H., et al., "Estimation of tissue hypothyroidism by a new clinical score: evaluation of patients with various grades of hypothyroidism and controls," *Journal of Clinical Endocrinology and Metabolism*, 1997 Mar.; 82(3): 771–776. (Clinical signs reflect hypothyroidism better than blood T4 and TSH levels.)

Chapter 6:

Dolidze, N.M., Kezeli, D.D.F., et al. Changes in intra- and extracellular Ca2+ concentration and prostaglandin E2 synthesis in osteoblasts of the femoral bone in experimental hyper- and hypothyroidism. *Bulletin of Experimental Biology and Medicine*, 2007 Jul;144(1):17–20. National Institute of Health, Vital Health Statistics.

Chapter 7:

DeCava, J., *The Real Truth about Vitamins and Anti-oxidants*, Health Science Series #5, a Printery, West Yarmouth, MA, 1997.

Kabara, J., *Fats Are Good for You and Other Secrets*, North Atlantic Books, Berkley, CA, 2008.

Chapter 8:

Barnes, K., *10 Best Ways to Manage Stress*, Take Charge Books, Brevard, NC 2013.

Carpi, MN, et al., "Stress: It's worse than you think," *Psychology Today*, Jan., 1996.

Karlamangla, A., et al., "Increase in epinephrine excretion is associated with cognitive decline in elderly men: MacArthur studies of successful aging," *Psychoneuroendocrinology*, 2005: 30(5):453–460.

Tsolaki, M., et al., "Severe psychological stress in elderly individuals: a proposed model of neurodegeneration and its implications," *American Journal of Alzheimer's Disease and Other Dementia*, 2009; 24(2):85–94.

Virtanen, M., et al. "Long working hours and cognitive function: The Whitehall II Study," *American Journal of Epidemiology*, 2009: 169:596–605.

Chapter 9:

Bond A, Alavi A et al. The relationship between exposed galactose and N-acetylglucosamine residues on IgG in rheumatoid arthritis (RA), juvenile chronic arthritis (JCA) and Sjögren's syndrome (SS). *Clinical and Experimental Immunology* 1996 Jul;105(1):99–103.

Panzironi C, Silvestroni N et al. An increase in the carbohydrate moiety of alpha 2-macroglobulin is associated with systemic lupus erythematosus (SLE). *Biochemistry and Molecular Biology International* 1997 Dec;43(6):1305–22.

Bond A, Alavi A et al. A detailed lectin analysis of IgG glycosylation, demonstrating disease specific changes in terminal galactose and N-acetylglucosamine. *Journal of Autoimmunology* 1997 Feb;10(1);77–85.

Aspartame: www.mercola.com/article/aspartame/weight_gain_myth.htm.

According to an article in *Technology Review*, "aspartame may actually stimulate appetite and bring on a craving for carbohydrates" (Farber 52). An article in *Utne Reader* claims, "researchers believe that any kind of sweet taste signals body cells to store carbohydrates and fats, which in turn causes the body to crave more food" (Lamb 16). From the San Francisco Chronicle, Jean Weininger states that "studies have shown that people who use artificial sweeteners don't necessarily reduce their consumption of sugar—or their total calorie intake. . . . Having a diet soda makes it okay to eat a double cheeseburger and a chocolate mousse pie" (1/ZZ1). "The American Cancer Society (1986) documented the fact that persons using artificial sweeteners gain more weight than those who avoid them" (Roberts 150).

Mathias B, Hoffmann, K et al. Dietary pattern, inflammation, and incidence of type 2 diabetes in women. *American Journal of Clinical Nutrition* 2005.

Liang Y, Maier V et al. The effect of artificial sweetener on insulin secretion. II. Stimulation of insulin release from isolated rat islets by Acesulfame K (in vitro experiments). *Hormones and Metabolic Resistance* 1987 Jul;19(7):285–9.

Stellman SD and Garfinkel L. Patterns of artificial sweetener use and weight change in an American Cancer Society prospective study. *Appetite* 1988;11 Suppl 1:85–91. (This is the seminal study in this field).

www.webmd.com/diet/news/20050613/drink-more-diet-soda-gain-more-weight.

(This scientific data was presented to the American Diabetes Association in 2005 by researchers from the University of Texas—lead researcher Sharon Fowler—but no paper has ever been published.)

Index

About the Authors

Dr. Robert Thompson is a board-certified obstetrician and gynecologist who practices in Soldotna and Anchorage, Alaska. While he is technically a "women's doctor," his work to expose The Calcium Lie has brought him many patients who fall outside his specialty. In fact, now more than half of his patients come to him for nutrition counseling and many of them have found long-term relief from chronic disease, including obesity, diabetes, hypothyroidism and adrenal fatigue. He happily counts among his patients many men and children as well as women who seek out his assistance as a gynecologist as well as a nutrition specialist.

He received his medical training at the University of Kentucky and has practiced in California, Pennsylvania, Hawaii and Alaska.

Dr. Thompson lives in Soldotna, Alaska, with his three labs, Ruger, Mys-tika and Zack, where he takes great delight in fly fishing, hunting, hiking, canoeing, water and snow skiing, snow machining, playing concert violin and raising and training Labrador retrievers.

Kathleen Barnes is a widely traveled journalist with more than 35 years of experience in publishing, print and broadcast media. In recent years she has specialized in medical, health and sustainable living for national magazines and newspapers and as author, coauthor and editor of more than 15 books.

She has lived in Europe, Asia and Africa and brings a broad international perspective to her writing.

Kathleen lives in the mountains of western North Carolina with her husband, Joe, and three dogs, one cat and two horses.